LIVING HEADACHE FREE

Headaches are a complex and incompletely understood affliction. Recent advancements in the field have improved the understanding of this disorder. Medical treatments now provide relief by addressing the headache process rather than merely symptom control. Days of disability due to sudden headache attacks are becoming unnecessary for millions of headache sufferers.

As a chronic disorder, headaches are more than a series of acute attacks that, improperly attended, cause significant disability. Managing the chronic nature of this disorder requires a cooperative partnership with the medical system and personal motivation to be an involved participant in headache care.

Today is a hopeful time for those who have spent years being disabled by headaches. Perhaps even more exciting is a future of living more headache-free.

HEADACHE FREE

ROGER CADY, M.D.

KATHLEEN FARMER, Psy. D.

Foreword by C. Norman Shealy, M.D., Ph.D.

Illustrations by Jackie Aher

BANTAM BOOKS
NEW YORK   TORONTO   LONDON
SYDNEY   AUCKLAND

HEADACHE FREE

A Bantam Book / published by arrangement
with the authors

PUBLISHING HISTORY
Moray Press edition published 1993
Bantam edition / January 1996

Grateful acknowledgment is made to Scott C. Farmer for the
original artwork upon which the drawings in this book were based.

In Canada *Aspirin* is a registered trademark
owned by Sterling Winthrop Inc.

ISBN 0-553-57000-5

Published simultaneously in the United States and Canada

Bantam Books are published by Bantam Books, a division of Bantam
Doubleday Dell Publishing Group, Inc. Its trademark, consisting of the
words "Bantam Books" and the portrayal of a rooster, is Registered in
U.S. Patent and Trademark Office and in other countries. Marca
Registrada. Bantam Books, 1540 Broadway, New York, New York 10036.

PRINTED IN THE UNITED STATES OF AMERICA
OPM   0 9 8 7 6

DISCLAIMER

This book is intended to be an informational source for headache sufferers. The authors and the publisher are not engaged in rendering medical advice on diagnosis and treatment of headaches. The guidelines presented are the opinions of the authors but any medical diagnosis or therapy should be directed and supervised by an individual's physician.

The case studies presented are actual reports from headache patients, but their names and some details have been changed to protect confidentiality.

To our fathers,
Kenneth and John,
who passed on a legacy
of innovation and independence.

ACKNOWLEDGMENTS

We wish to thank those headache sufferers who have agreed to let us tell their stories. Their experiences will help others cope with disabling headaches.

We are indebted to our families, who offered support, encouragement and understanding. Without them, we would still only be talking and dreaming.

We are also grateful to the staff of the Shealy Institute for their opinions, time and interest. We extend special thanks to Colleen Baker, Deni Carruth, Marvin Roberts, Ken Everett, Mariann Burnetti-Atwell, Kay Lund, Barbara Hall and Kim Kitterman for posing for photographs and suggesting exercises.

Dr. C. Norman Shealy too occupies an important place in our hearts as a valuable source of inspiration and knowledge.

We are likewise indebted to the second grade class of Greenwood Laboratory School for the drawings of "how a headache feels."

Thanks also to Charles Farmer for his editorial suggestions.

FOREWORD

Headache is one of the most debilitating of all disorders, often robbing its sufferers of much of the quality of life. Major advances in headache management in the past two decades offer hope, for the first time in history, to a majority of headache sufferers. Pharmacological and nonpharmacological treatment alternatives, such as new medications, biofeedback training, cranial electrical stimulation and photostimulation, provide relief. Recognition of subtle precipitating factors can prevent chronic daily headache, inappropriate medication and medication abuse.

Thus physicians, patients and their families and friends can benefit from the simple and very wise advice presented in this book. Its authors have become leading proponents of comprehensive headache management. Significantly, Dr. Cady is a headache specialist and a board certified family physician. Since there are ten times as many family physicians as there are neurologists, it is critical that competent headache management become the *standard* of care among primary physicians.

This book serves two valuable purposes. First, it provides a comprehensive overview of headache and its proper management. More importantly, it provides a personal experiential method for self-regulation. Ultimately, *you* are responsible for assuring yourself of competent care. This book provides the framework for achieving that goal.

The good news is that, of all the pain problems presented to physicians and pain clinics, headaches are the *most successfully* treated problems seen—if the principles laid down are followed. I commend the authors on this great contribution to your welfare. And I commend you for making the effort, well worthwhile, required to control headaches.

C. Norman Shealy, M.D., Ph.D.
Founder, Shealy Institute and the
American Holistic Medical Association

CONTENTS

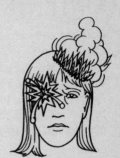

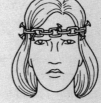

Once Upon a Time

I used to have headaches only once a month, right before my period, when my mind doesn't seem to work. I'd have to spend 1 or 2 days in bed. I'd get rest and I'd never plan anything around that time of the month.

But then my headaches became more frequent. I'd have to take 4 aspirin at a time, and then 6. I started to get them once a week. My boss didn't mind my being off once a month, but once a week was too much.

As a receptionist-secretary, I was constantly interrupted throughout the day. I usually took typing home, catching up after dinner and before bedtime to prevent facing an overload the next day. As a mother of two small children (ages 2 and 4), I spent as much time as I could with them, but that was never enough. At home I felt much like I did at work, pressured, frustrated and not good enough to meet all the expectations of boss, kids and husband. As the wife of a self-employed painter, I wanted to be supportive to Jim, my husband. But the demands of work, home and children left little for me to give Jim and nothing for myself.

My brother reminded me that Mother used to have headaches until she had her long hair cut short. Even though Jim treasured my long straight blond hair and didn't want me to trim it, my family warned that all that hair was heavy and a strain on the scalp. "No wonder you have headaches," they'd tell me.

My best friend, Yvonne, had a cousin whose headaches disappeared when she separated from her husband. Yvonne suggested that I have a serious talk with Jim. My brother-in-law, Fred, told me that some strong medicine would knock out my headache.

Everyone seemed to have a different opinion; everyone knew someone who tried something different to get rid of headaches. Since the headaches used to oc-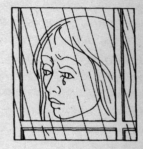cur before my peri- ods, my mother-in-law recommended an ap- pointment with a gyne- cologist to talk about a hysterectomy. "After all, you don't plan to have any more children, do you?" she asked. A neighbor's uncle had head- aches and now has a brain tumor. The grocery checkout girl pointed out that her headaches re- solved when her "bad back" was treated.

I was bewildered, frightened and desperate by the time I asked for help with my headaches. I was also drinking 6 cups of coffee in the morning and 4 to 6 cans of diet pop in the afternoon. I ate Oriental food for lunch twice a week and snacked on a chocolate bar daily during break.

After a complete medical examination, I braced myself for the worst possible news. But, to my sur- prise, the recommendations were simple and straightforward. I was advised to eliminate caffeine and diet pop, to eat regular meals and avoid monosodium glutamate (MSG), and maintain a regular sleep pattern.

To help me manage a stressful lifestyle, I was encouraged to see a psychologist. The psychologist taught me biofeedback techniques and relaxation methods. I also learned that I cannot be all things to all people, and that I needed to pace myself and say "no" to excessive demands. I was given medication to prevent headaches from occurring during my menstrual cycle and another medicine to help stop the headaches when they occur. Overall, I was reassured that I am healthy. Also I learned simple ways to manage the headaches.

12 Myths About Headache Sufferers

MYTH #1:
Recurrent headaches mean I have a psychological problem.

MYTH #2:
Headaches are something I have to learn to live with. There is no help.

MYTH #3:
The only way to stop my headaches is to stop living. Headaches have taken over my life.

MYTH #4:
Recurrent headaches are not serious. After all, it's just a headache.

MYTH #5:
My children will suffer headaches because I do.

MYTH #6:
Medication is the only relief for my headaches.

MYTH #7:
Recurrent headaches mean that I am more likely to have a stroke, tumor or other brain disorder.

MYTH #8:
My headaches are caused by my neck being out-of-line.

MYTH #9:
Severe headaches must be migraines.

MYTH #10:
Recurrent headaches are a female disorder.

MYTH #11:
Headaches are an excuse for getting out of doing what I don't want to do.

MYTH #12:
Headaches are not worth the time and expense of seeing a doctor.

HEADACHE FREE

1

DEMYSTIFYING HEADACHE

From a boiling cauldron of myth and misunderstanding, the mysteries of headaches are beginning to unravel and find a place in scientific understanding. Fears of demons and devils are being calmed by scientific facts. The secrets of this ancient plague are being unlocked and, today, there is new hope and assistance for headache sufferers.

Headaches cause personal suffering, disrupt families and interfere with work and leisure. Striking unpredictably, an attack shatters a sense of self-control. Medications are often less than effective or produce unwanted side effects.

Present day myths about headaches often induce a sense of isolation, shame and helplessness. Before healing can begin, the headache sufferer needs to know that headaches are a treatable and significant disorder. Psychological conflicts are generally the result, not the cause, of chronic headaches.

Fortunately, the seeds of change are sprouting. Recent advances in research are expanding the medical community's understanding of headache and creating treatments that work. Headache sufferers have more options for effective control of symptoms through their own efforts. More than doctor visits and drugs, the management of headache involves understanding the headache problem, identifying factors that precipitate headaches and working with medical providers in a therapeutic partnership.

Truths About Headache Sufferers

Myth #1: Recurrent headaches mean I have a psychological problem.

Fact: Headaches are the result of biochemical changes in the brain. Stress, acting on the nervous system, makes headaches more likely to occur. The stress may be chemical, emotional, biological or psychological. Psychological problems can arise from poorly managed headaches but, for the most part, psychological problems do not cause headaches.

Myth #2: Headaches are something I have to learn to live with. There is no help.

Fact: Headaches can be managed, not cured. With proper medical care, education and effort, almost all headache sufferers can reduce the pain and disability of headaches.

Myth #3: The only way to stop my headaches is to stop living. Headaches have taken over my life.

Fact: Frequent disabling headaches occur in an unpredictable fashion and create fear of the next headache attack. As headache frequency increases, the greater the fear grows. This can lead to a vicious cycle where anticipation of the next headache becomes the stress that generates more headaches. Proper headache management, addressing medical care and lifestyle, can break this cycle and restore control.

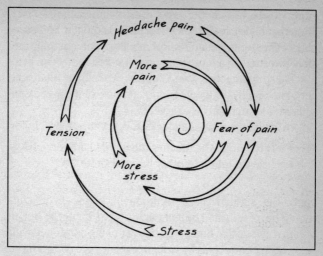

The Vicious Spiral of Headache

Myth #4: Recurrent headaches are not serious. After all, it's just a headache.

Fact: Most headaches are not life-threatening but may seriously influence an individual's quality of life and coping abilities. They strain family life, disrupt leisure activity and diminish career opportunities.

Myth #5: My children will suffer headaches because I do.

Fact: Children learn how to deal with stress from the behaviors of their parents. Research suggests that the threshold of handling incoming stimuli to the brain may be inherited (see Chapter 3). By learning how to manage stress effectively, however, children experience coping alternatives which will boost their resistance to headaches.

Myth #6: Medication is the only relief for my headaches.

Fact: Headaches are the result of many interacting factors. There is no simple answer. Medication is often a necessary part of headache treatment, but rarely is it the complete answer. Some medications when used too frequently can actually cause headaches (see Chapter 4). Optimal headache care almost always involves participation of the headache sufferer and medical care provider.

Myth #7: Recurrent headaches mean that I am more likely to have a stroke, tumor or other brain disorder.

Fact: The sudden onset of frequent, severe headaches should be investigated by a physician (see Chapter 4). But research suggests that heavy cigarette smoking combined with using birth control pills by women over the age of 30 is more predictive of the possibility of a stroke than the occurrence of headaches. Brain tumors are a rare cause of headaches.

Myth #8: My headaches are caused by my neck being out-of-line.

Fact: The status of the neck needs to be medically evaluated because headache pain may originate with neck and back problems. Pain during headaches, however, is often projected or referred to the neck and shoulders. Usually, tension in the neck is the result, not the cause, of a headache.

Myth #9: Severe headaches must be migraines.

Fact: There are many different types of headaches. The diagnosis of most headaches rests solely on the medical history because there are no tests that substantiate the diagnosis. Severe headaches should be diagnosed by a physician to begin proper treatment.

Myth #10: Recurrent headaches are a female disorder.

Fact: Migraines are influenced by hormonal factors. This is reflected in the fact that 3 times more women than men have migraines. Six percent of adult men suffer from migraines, however, and studies show that the disability is not influenced by gender.

Myth #11: Headaches are an excuse for getting out of doing what I don't want to do.

Fact: Headaches can be a serious disabling illness. Quality of life studies of those with migraine demonstrate greater impairment of lifestyle than with most other chronic illnesses. There are more benign ways to avoid undesired activity than with headaches.

Myth #12: Headaches are not worth the time and expense of seeing a doctor.

Fact: Not managing headaches is far more costly than caring for them. Each year the average headache sufferer loses time and income due to headache disability. These losses exceed the cost of quality medical treatment.

Based on scientific findings, *Headache Free* instructs those with headaches on how to construct an individualized headache management program. The

HEADACHES CAN BE A GUIDE TO SELF-UNDERSTANDING.

headache sufferer becomes an integral part of therapy.

This book emphasizes solutions. Chapters explore different dimensions of headaches and provide measures for self-assessment. Lifestyles may need adjustment to alter the headache pattern.

Ultimately, headaches can be used as a guide to self-understanding. Stresses that promote headaches can often be modified, promoting a sense of control and enhancing the quality of an individual's life. The good news is that headaches are manageable and now is the time to begin.

2

A BRIEF HISTORY
OF HEADACHE

A Migraine Day

It's out there . . . like a freight train in a far-away dream. Almost unconsciously, I stir in my sleep and awaken. No, this can't be. Not today. I quickly slip out of bed to swallow some medicine. No, it can't be today. There just isn't time. Maybe if I sleep; maybe the medicine will take hold and I can avoid this terrible headache. . . . Prayers are not answered. My stomach is queasy. The pain begins to throb. Even the first rays of morning sun are unwelcome. Yes, today is going to be a migraine day.

So the story goes. Sufferers throughout time have been caught in fear of a disabling headache. Relief is elusive, just out of reach. The search for a solution, though relentless, continues today.

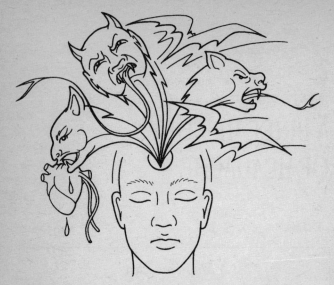

Trepanning, a surgical procedure performed in early times, was thought to release demons from the head and cure a severe headache.

Trepanning

Even before recorded history, humankind was in pursuit of an effective treatment for headaches. Archaeologists have found skulls, dating as far back as 7000 B.C., which have been cut with stone knives, opening the top of the head. Called trepanning, this surgical procedure is perhaps the oldest known treatment for headaches. Trepanning was devised to release demons and evil spirits presumed to reside in the skull and cause headaches. Except in South America, where cocaine was used, this procedure was done without the aid of an anesthetic. Yet, an estimated 50 percent of people survived. Trepanning was recommended as a treatment for intractable headaches as late as 1630 by the eminent British physician William Harvey.

Greek and Roman Remedies

The Greeks offered headache sufferers herbal remedies, representing early attempts at pharmacological treatment. An especially exotic method used the torpedo fish, native to the Mediterranean Sea. Applied to the head, this fish delivered a stout electric shock, much like an electric eel. The shock reportedly alleviated head pain.

The Greeks believed that an evil deity named "Kreves" entered the body through the intestinal tract and elaborated a humour that resulted in a headache. Therapies often induced vomiting to rid the body of this evil deity and of head pain.

Within the Roman Empire many of the Greek treatments for headaches continued to be practiced. As Christianity spread and became a dominant influence on health practices, pain was considered atonement or penance for sin. In fact, the word *pain* is derived from the Latin word *poena*, which translates as punishment.

Even today, many individuals believe that a headache is punishment or a sign of weakness. In fact, a cultural bias traditionally classifies headaches as the result of an inability to cope effectively with life. Such a misunderstanding hinders adequate headache management because people often feel ashamed or guilty for admitting that they are afflicted with headaches.

> *POENA* IS LATIN FOR PAIN AND MEANS TO PUNISH.

Primitive Cures

Prayers and incantations have been sung and chanted throughout the ages as attempts to relieve headaches. Early Polynesians believed so strongly in the power of their god of headache that they evoked the god to attack their enemies

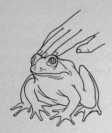

A bullfrog, rubbed on the head, helps relieve a headache, according to folklore.

before battle, giving their army the advantage of being head-ache-free.

Certain cultures believed that a headache occurred if a bird used a strand of hair in building its nest. Folklore advised wearing the boiled nest of a swallow around the neck for 3 days to relieve a headache. Mexicans rubbed the headache away using a live toad or bullfrog, applied to the site of discomfort.

American Indians offered headache sufferers several remedies, including tobacco, willow bark and a concoction of beaver testes. These therapies probably provided relief because the nicotine of tobacco constricts blood vessels and the willow bark and beaver testes contain aspirin-like chemicals.

Quackery

Desperate headache sufferers have been targets for con artists and quacks. Throughout Europe during the sixteenth century, a popular scam was to surgically remove "head stones." The unscrupulous surgeon would make an incision into the scalp and "remove" a small white stone which had been given to the surgeon during the operation by an assistant.

"Every time I plan something, I get a headache and have to cancel out. It never fails."

A ninth-century British "cure" suggested that one should drink a concoction of the juice of elder seeds, cow's brain, goat dung and vinegar to relieve headaches. There is little evidence that this mixture had any effect on a headache.

In the late 1600s, the grandfather of Charles Darwin suggested that those with headaches should be placed on a centrifuge that would drive blood from the head into the feet. Though this was based on the prevailing scientific thought of the day, centrifuging someone during the throes of a severe headache would likely border on torture.

Throughout early American history, traveling medicine men sold tonics and tinctures that promised to cure headaches. The main ingredient in many of these concoctions was alcohol or cocaine, both of which provoke headaches. Devices, too, were peddled as cures. Tight bands around the head, electric shocks and even X rays were all reported to stop headaches.

Basically, there is no cure for headaches, even though a variety of methods may bring relief. Effective headache control is a matter of learning how best to manage head pain by individualizing treatment approaches.

Early Scientific Explanations

Science reflects the underlying beliefs of the culture and is an attempt to interpret the mysteries of life and nature. Headaches, even today, remain a puzzle. Early explanations revolved around the belief that evil spirits produced a headache as a result of sin. During the Renaissance, science discounted these mystic beliefs and began to explore illness on a more rational basis.

Thomas Willis, the father of modern-day neurology, was the first to suggest that migraine pain was a disorder of blood vessels. Because migraine is a disorder affecting more women than men and is associated with menses, he hypothesized that channels connected the uterus with the brain and elaborated a toxin, causing blood vessel changes. This offered no explanation for migraines in men.

Sigmund Freud, the father of psychoanalysis, suffered from headaches. He was the first to suggest, however, that physical symptoms may be an expression of unconscious conflict. Freud invented the "talking cure" to encourage the individual to bring forgotten traumas into awareness. Through the process of resolving the problem, the physical symptoms became unnecessary.

Later on, followers of the psychodynamic theory expounded the idea that headaches, especially in women, were commonly due to emotional problems. Often grouped under the catchword of hysteria, the symptoms of headaches were dismissed as imaginary and hormonally related. Interestingly, the Greek root of hysteria is *husterikos,* meaning womb.

These biases remain common in medicine today. Hormonal influences are frequently believed to disrupt thinking. And migraine is often thought of as a woman's disease. Though changes in mood and thought can occur whenever the balance of the body is disrupted, it is important to keep in mind that changes in the female reproductive system are normal and healthy.

"My headaches are like the boogeyman. I'm really afraid of them."

Edward Living believed that headaches represented changes in the electrical and chemical nature of the brain. He referred to migraines as "brain seizures," laying the foundation for the modern neurogenic theory of headaches. He further understood that control of headaches could be enhanced by proper health habits.

Many factors may contribute to an imbalance in the nervous system, producing physical symptoms, such as a headache. The body utilizes counterbalancing internal mechanisms to restore functioning. The desire of the body to balance itself is called *homeostasis,* a process that can be assisted by personal health choices.

Windows to Creativity

Throughout human history, certain headache sufferers have enhanced their lives and creative genius through their unique experiences with headaches. For instance, approximately 15 percent of migraineurs experience aura prior to the onset of their headache. Auras usually consist of visual disturbances (flashing lights, blinking stars, zigzag patterns of light and dark, changes in visual acuity) or tingling around the lips or in the fingers of one hand. At times, however, auras can cause spectacular neurological disturbances, such as hallucinations. At first, migraineurs with auras may believe that they are going blind, have a life-threatening illness or their sanity is crumbling. Some migraineurs, however, have been able to incorporate these periodic changes in perception into creativity.

One example is the twelfth-century mystic, Hildegard, who understood her aura to represent deeper meaning. Believing these experiences to be divinely inspired, she transformed her visions into pieces of art, music and man-

Fortification spectra, kaleidoscopic patterns resembling a fort, are sometimes seen during a migraine aura.

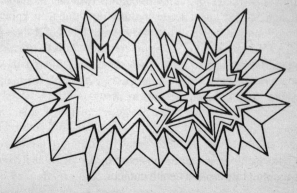

uscripts. Lewis Carroll, too, interpreted auras as windows to creativity. His extraordinary auras distorted space and time and influenced the characters and happenings in his books, *Alice in Wonderland* and *Through the Looking Glass*.

Thomas Jefferson and Ulysses S. Grant also suffered from headaches. History records that General Grant had struggled through a sleepless night, enduring a severe headache, when a messenger arrived at his tent with a message from General Robert E. Lee. After General Grant read the letter, which announced Lee's surrender, his headache miraculously disappeared.

Charles Darwin, Virginia Woolf, Edgar Allan Poe and George Bernard Shaw were agonized by headaches throughout their lives. Their genius outdistanced the drain of periodic attacks. In fact, by not knowing when the next episode will strike, the present moment can hold special value and drive the individual to pursue as much of life as possible.

Even in modern times, headaches have been a powerful force, affecting such outstanding athletes as tennis star Chris Evert and basketball legend Kareem Abdul-Jabbar.

Ironically, the more preoccupied with pain a headache sufferer becomes, the larger the disability grows. At times, a headache can consume everything else. But with knowledge, learning the tools to prevent headaches and finding ways to ameliorate the suffering, control returns to the individual. Confidence swells. Living becomes fun again. A headache means a time to reconsider methods for maintaining calm, balance and perspective.

Headaches Today

A headache is as misunderstood today as it has been throughout the ages. Minor headaches are experienced by almost everyone at some time. Yet these headaches are

Headache Control

I was born with headaches. They have been with me as long as I can remember. For years I felt that they were just a part of life. They interfered with my dreams and I felt as if I were damaged. No one seemed to understand. I went to dozens of doctors, tried a pharmacy of different medicines and underwent countless tests; yet the headache continued to run my life. I often found myself helpless and depressed.

One day I met a friend who had headaches very similar to mine and who invited me to a headache support group. Suddenly, I discovered that I was not alone. I learned a lot about headaches and how I could control them, rather than they controlling me. I learned that there were medications that could help and how to use them properly. I learned that many things in my diet and lifestyle made headaches more likely. I decided that I could learn to manage headaches.

My doctor suggested I learn biofeedback. I saw a psychologist who taught me to manage my life more effectively and I learned to do biofeedback. I soon had better control of my headaches.

I practice that control every day. I still get occasional headaches, but I have medication that controls them. Most importantly, I no longer live in fear of the next headache. I feel that after all these years, I'm in control of my headaches and my life.

much different than the severe head pain endured by many headache sufferers. Severe headaches are a serious disorder. While not fatal, a headache disables its victim and causes considerable torment and hardship. Affecting the entire body, severe or frequent headaches can temporarily halt one's life. This process disrupts families, careers and robs society of the possible contributions from the headache sufferer.

Headaches of this nature affect 1 in 11 adult Americans and their prevalence has increased over 60 percent through the last decade. The reason for this dramatic increase is unknown, but many speculate that pollutants, diet and the increasing demands of daily life are likely factors.

Headaches are very disabling, causing an estimated 150 million days to be lost to the American workforce. The average migraine sufferer loses 13 work days and 8 days of leisure time per year to attacks. Efficiency, too, lessens as people try to work with a headache. Over time, decreased work productivity and absenteeism can add up to missed promotions, less pay or lost jobs.

Frequent headaches can interfere with family life. The fear of bringing on another attack can prevent a person from making plans with family and friends. Guilt and despair often result. Family members feel helpless or, at times, angry because they do not understand the headache process and feel powerless to intervene.

"With a headache, everything is doom and gloom; will I ever get better?"

Headaches are underdiagnosed; less than one-half of female migraineurs and less than one-third of male migraineurs have been diagnosed by a physician even though they suffer headaches that interfere with daily living.

Headaches are undertreated; there is inadequate information available to headache sufferers about how to manage headaches. At the same time, medication that assists the headache sufferer is underutilized; most individuals rely on over-the-counter medications.

HEADACHES ARE UNDER-DIAGNOSED AND UNDER-TREATED.

Medical providers may not appreciate the complexity of the headache process and the nonpharmacologic treatment approaches useful in headache management.

Social and medical biases about headaches abound. Headache sufferers are often viewed with suspicion by employers and medical personnel. Headaches are frequently the subject of jokes and often seen as a weakness or the inability to cope with stress. Headaches are viewed as a fact of life, a condition for which there is little to be done. Often, attempts to seek treatment are ineffective. Long waits in an emergency department, innuendos of seeking drugs, numerous expensive medical evaluations and treatments that are less than effective or disabling are all too frequent encounters for the headache sufferer.

Yet medical science is revealing some of the secrets of the headache process. Many specialists in the field of headaches have proposed more comprehensive approaches to this disorder. Headache sufferers are encouraged to take an active part in the headache treatment process. More effective, safer and better tolerated medications are being developed. There is a greater emphasis on treating the process of headaches rather than numbing the brain against pain. Individualizing a management style with each headache sufferer who works as a partner with medical personnel to better control a headache is becoming the model of effective treatment. There is new hope for the headache sufferer.

3

THE HEADACHE SPECTRUM

Headaches can be big or little, frequent or infrequent, disabling or minor. Headaches can warn of another disease or be a disorder unto themselves. Even in the same individual, several different headaches can be present. In most cases, a headache is the disorder rather than a symptom of an underlying disease. The spectrum of headaches touches the lives of almost everyone; some through personal experience, others through the headache's impact. Through understanding, the mystery of headaches unravels and a management scheme evolves aimed at controlling, even preventing, much of the misery of headaches.

Why Do Headaches Occur?

Science does not yet completely understand why people suffer headaches or why different types of headaches occur. Headaches occur sometime in life for almost everyone. Genetics seem to play a significant role in predicting susceptibility to migraine and tension headaches. Ultimately, however, headaches arise from the interaction between genetic vulnerability and the environment.

If a person is born with the genetic predisposition for migraines and lives in a migraine-prone environment, migraines will likely emerge. If, on the other hand, the genetic predisposition of tension headaches is dominant, then tension headaches are likely to evolve. Other headaches, such as cluster, do not appear to have a significant genetic component, but are affected by the environment.

Serotonin: Serotonin is a brain chemical that plays an important role in preventing headaches. Serotonin is a neurotransmitter, a chemical used by the nerves for communication. Secreted from the nerve ending when the nerve is stimulated, serotonin moves to a special target area called a receptor. The neurochemical and receptor act much like a molecular lock and key. When linked together, this neurochemical-receptor interaction unlocks a specific response.

Receptors throughout the body interact with serotonin. Some are in the intestinal tract, others are in certain blood cells and many different types are in nerve tissue. Depending on which pathways are activated, serotonin can initiate a wide variety of responses. In addi-

"Life would be perfect if I didn't have these headaches. I love my husband and two sons. I've had to work since they were born, but they value the quality time we share as much as I do. My older son is 28, lives at home and is still looking for a job. My husband takes the boat out every weekend and fishes for bass. Sometimes he takes one of the boys. I don't go because I don't like water: I can't swim. My job is stressful, but I handle the pressure fine."

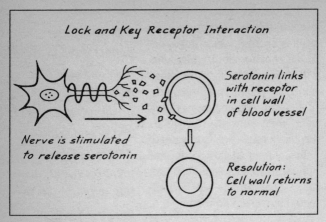

Receptor Interaction with Serotonin

tion to its role in a headache, serotonin modulates sleep, mood, sexual behavior, blood vessel activity and other important functions.

Serotonin levels change significantly before and during

Headache Resolution

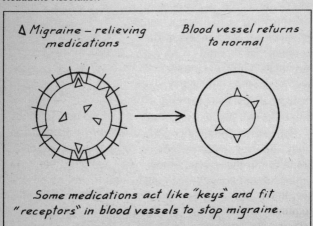

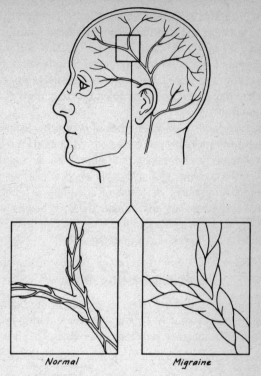

Normal   *Migraine*

Blood Vessels in Migraine (Magnified)

many headaches. In a migraine, as serotonin levels change, the brain loses its ability to regulate certain blood vessels in the head. These blood vessels expand and the liquid part of the blood leaks into the surrounding tissue. The body responds by releasing chemicals that cause inflammation (similar to what happens in allergic reactions or arthritis). The affected area of the blood vessel becomes very irritated. As blood is pumped through, the irritated blood vessels stretch and a person feels the throbbing pain of a migraine.

During the migraine process, serotonin levels drop. Some

of the drugs that relieve migraine mimic the action of serotonin by fitting into certain serotonin receptor sites where nerves and blood vessels communicate. This shrinks the blood vessel and reverses the painful inflammatory response. When activated in this manner, the nerve fibers that carry the pain message to the brain become more difficult to stimulate.

The mechanism of other types of headaches is less understood but probably involve serotonin. Perhaps serotonin helps the body maintain equilibrium. With accumulated stresses, the nervous system's capacity to adjust becomes impaired. Temporarily deprived of adequate neurochemicals to make necessary adjustments, the body begins to lose its ability to adapt and a headache results. The body needs time and space to rest and regenerate.

Headache Threshold

The headache threshold refers to an area of the brain that helps the body maintain chemical balance during periods of change. This balance is called *homeostasis*. The threshold

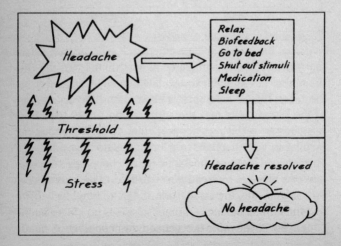

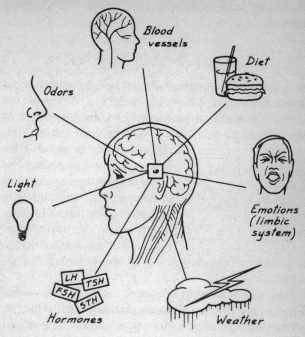

Blood vessels

Diet

Odors

Light

Emotions (limbic system)

LH TSH
FSH
STH
Hormones

Weather

Relay Station

monitors the body's relationship to the internal and external environment. With connections to other parts of the brain, the threshold acts as a switchboard, receiving information from the limbic system, where emotions are registered, from the hypothalamus, where hormones are regulated, from the cortex, where thoughts and fears are remembered, and from the muscles of the head and neck. Occurrences in the environment, such as chemicals from our diet or a change in the weather, can also impact on this relay station. When the circuits fill up, the system bogs down and the normal balance—homeostasis—is no longer maintained. For those with the genetic susceptibility to headaches, the change in chemical balance may lead to a head-ache.

Learning About My Threshold

Many individuals control headaches by learning about their unique sensitivities. A diary is a useful tool to pinpoint the factors that lead to a headache. The diary keeps track of diet, weather, sleep, mealtimes and day-to-day stress. Menstrual fluctuations are also important. Unusual events need to be recorded, too. See yourself as an explorer discovering how you and your environment interact. Try to detect the environment that spawns headaches. Ask family members to help, as they may be aware of things that are not readily apparent.

> YOU ARE AN EXPLORER DISCOVERING HOW YOU AND YOUR ENVIRONMENT INTERACT.

Hundreds of different influences can precipitate a headache. Occasionally, a single factor, such as a certain food like red wine or aged cheese, may cause a headache. It is then called a *headache trigger*. More often a combination of precipitating events add up to a headache. Learning to avoid these factors will boost immunity to headaches.

There are buffers for the headache threshold as well. These include learning to cope more effectively with stress, getting adequate sleep and enjoying a period of relaxation twice a day. Some medications also enhance the threshold's resistance to headache precipitators. By living a predictable lifestyle and nurturing health, a headache-protective environment is created.

Are Tension–type Headaches and Migraines Different?

Tension–type headaches and migraines may share funda-mental similarities, but at the same time, have unique differ-ences. Historically, the explanation of the pain in a tension headache is related to excessive tightness within muscles of the head and neck. In a migraine, the pain is presumed to arise from blood vessels. This distinction, however, is not al-ways precise. For example, in migraines it is common to have significant tenderness of muscles during the attack.

Today, most headache specialists suggest that the initiat-ing events of both migraines and tension–type headaches originate in the brain. These headaches become differenti-ated because separate nerve pathways are activated during the assault of stressors acting on the nervous system. When pathways from the muscles are activated, a tension–type headache results; if those from blood vessels are aroused, then a migraine strikes. Of course, activation of several dif-ferent pathways can occur, producing an overlap of symp-toms called *mixed headaches*.

Tension-Migraine Pathways

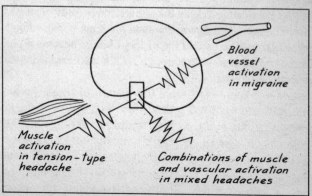

Blood vessel activation in migraine

Muscle activation in tension–type headache

Combinations of muscle and vascular activation in mixed headaches

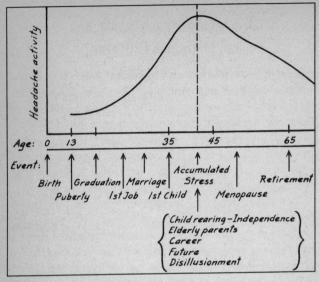

Life Cycle of Headache

The Life Cycle of Headaches

Headaches typically begin in childhood or adolescence and increase in frequency through the 30s and 40s. During years of headache activity, the quality and severity of attacks may change. Often major events in life may increase headache activity. The natural life history of most headache patterns, however, increases through midlife and declines with mature adulthood.

THE MORE OFTEN ONE HAS A HEADACHE, THE EASIER IT BECOMES TO ACTIVATE NERVE PATHWAYS THAT RESULT IN A HEADACHE.

This pattern of headache activity may relate to changes in the serotonin activity in the brain with maturity. Also, since many headaches are more common in women during times of hormonal changes, the postmenopause years, when hormone levels are stable, may produce less headache activity.

Headache Transformation

During the life cycle of headaches, the character of the attacks may change. Often headaches, like migraines, begin as discrete events with many headache-free days between attacks. As the pattern progresses, the attacks seem to blend together, producing a constant dull headache. Severe attacks may still strike and be disabling, but there is the addition of daily headache pain. Many important factors may transform headache episodes into more chronic patterns. By learning to minimize these factors, headache disability may be prevented.

Facilitation: The more often one has a headache, the easier it becomes to activate those nerve pathways that result in a headache. In other words, the threshold needed to trigger a headache is lowered. This process is called *facilitation* and may be initiated by many different factors, such as head or neck trauma, illness, poor posture, medications or simply experiencing frequent headaches. Facilitation underscores the need for early screening and control of headaches. Early intervention and treatment of headaches lessen the sensitivity of the nerve pathways and may prevent headaches from becoming chronic.

Medication: Improper use of certain medications may sensitize the headache threshold. These medications act as a catalyst to transform episodes of headache activity into a chronic daily headache problem. Ironically, these medications are initially effective in relieving headaches, but as their use becomes chronic, they actually perpetuate the headache process.

Rebound Headaches

I wouldn't have believed that my medication was causing my headaches. I thought it was time to find a new doctor. I had suffered with these headaches for years. Day in and day out, the headache would be there. The only medicine that helped me was Fiorinol. Sure, I was concerned about how much medicine I was using, but what else could I do?

My doctor suggested I attend a migraine support group meeting. I didn't want to go. It's not like I had been traumatized or was an alcoholic; I just had these headaches. But, after several weeks, I decided to go.

Members of the group understood right away what I was going through. A few had been in the same situation as I was. They told me that their doctor helped them get off the medication and how much better they felt. They no longer had headaches every day and their thinking had cleared. Once in a while they had headaches, but now medication worked and the headaches would disappear for weeks at a time. I thought, if they can do it, so can I.

The types of medication most often involved in this transformational process are pain medications, ergotamines, caffeine and medicine used to treat anxiety. These medications, when used on a daily or near-daily basis, create a type of chemical dependency. If the medication is abruptly terminated, a severe rebound headache occurs.

Caught in this cycle, the headache sufferer continues taking the medication to avoid a severe rebound headache. Over time, the medication becomes less effective at relieving the headache and a chronic headache pattern emerges.

"My headaches are snowballing and there is no way to stop them."

Over-the-counter headache medications, such as acetaminophen and aspirin, can initiate this cycle. Products which combine pain-relievers with caffeine are more potent inducers of headache transformation. Yet commercials advertise the safety and effectiveness of these headache products without pointing out that, with long-term daily use, they can worsen many headache patterns. Once

Headache Spiral

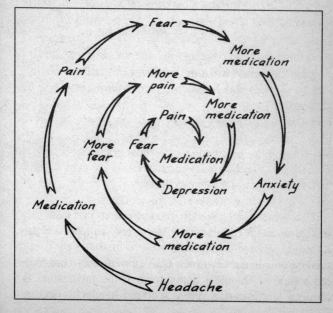

OVER-THE-COUNTER PAIN MEDICATION CAN PERPETUATE THE HEADACHE CYCLE.

this pattern has developed, medications useful in migraine prevention or treatment become less effective until the offending medication is stopped.

Modern View of Headaches

An understanding of headaches, though incomplete, has significantly advanced over the last few decades. Research delineating headache mechanisms has helped to validate headaches as a "real disorder." Advanced treatments are highly specific and very effective in rapidly relieving headache pain and disability.

Finding a Perspective for Your Headaches

Learning my headache pattern:
1) How old was I when my headaches began?
2) How often did headaches occur during the first few years?
3) Has the frequency or pattern of my headache activity changed?
4) Were there any significant events occurring in my life when this change occurred? Head or neck trauma? Emotional upset? Serious illness?
5) What medications do I use for headaches?
6) How much of each of these medications do I take?
7) How much caffeine do I use? (soda, coffee, chocolate, medication)
8) If I go without my medication, does a severe headache result?

If your answers suggest that your headaches are occurring more often, a transformation may be in progress. Headaches are a chronic disorder, but they do not necessarily have to worsen over time. Consult a physician and begin formulating a headache treatment plan.

Headache Diary

The Headache Diary is an invaluable ally in learning about yourself. Details about your life that are taken for granted are brought into awareness by writing down everyday happenings.

Instructions:
1. Make copies of the Headache Diary form, enough for one month.
2. Organize the Diary sheets in a loose-leaf notebook.
3. Review the Diary sheets every week and look for a pattern of events that lead to a headache.
4. Continue to refine the process by altering factors and measuring the body's response.

HEADACHE DIARY

Date_____ Hours of sleep last night_____ Quality of sleep_____

Medication taken_____
_____

	Excellent	Very Good	Good	Fair	Poor
My health today	1	2	3	4	5

What activities did I do today:
sports, work, fun, exercise, other?_____
_____

What activity did I have to eliminate due to
my physical health: sports, work, fun, exercise, other?_____
_____

	None	Mild	Moderate	Severe
Headache rating	0	1	2	3

How long did the pain last?_____

Method of relief_____

Location of the pain _____

Description of the pain_____

Symptoms associated with the headache_____
_____

What has the weather pattern been?_____

My feelings today were:

Happy energetic	Little uptight nervous	Downhearted worried or blue	Tired no energy	Hopeless helpless
1	2	3	4	5

Things I did, ate or drank that weren't good for me_____

Arguments I had _____

Unexpected events that happened to me_____

Worries or fears_____

Accomplishments _____

Something I will do tomorrow that will be a little different_____
_____

4

TYPES OF HEADACHES

A headache is not only painful, it is aggravating. The "why" behind the headache haunts the individual, generating fear. Realistically, there are no specific diagnostic tests for most headaches. Serious conditions can be excluded by medical investigation. But when the physician finds no underlying cause for headaches, the patient is often dismissed as having no "serious" problem even though headaches are ruining the person's life.

International Headache Society
Diagnostic Criteria

In 1988, the International Headache Society (IHS) composed a comprehensive guide for classifying headache and facial pain. This system standardized headache diagnosis for medical treatment and research; a migraine is a migraine is a migraine for physician, patient and researcher alike. Yet a headache may fulfill criteria for more than one headache diagnosis; the symptoms may change over time;

"At first I panicked because I thought I was going blind in the right eye. But then the sensation of someone pulling out my eye changed into a throbbing pain. After that first headache, I no longer felt relief over only having a migraine instead of being blind."

MIGRAINE, FRENCH
HĒMIKRANIA, GREEK
MIGRÄNE, GERMAN
MEGRIM, OLD ENGLISH

---

or the headache itself may transform from one type to another during a single episode.

Even though nearly 150 different headache diagnostic categories exist, the most common headache syndromes are migraine, tension, mixed, cluster, sinus, rebound and menstrual.

The single most important tool for evaluation of headaches is the person's medical history. Because no objective measurement of headaches exists, the essence of diagnosis rests in the individual's story.

Migraine

A migraine is not just a headache, but a disorder affecting the whole body. A migraine progresses through five distinct phases. Clearly defined attacks are separated by headache-free periods. Daily headaches are not migraines. Recognizing the spectrum of the entire process, a migraine sufferer can be alerted to cues prior to the onset of pain. By altering behaviors and using medication properly, the pain and disability may be diverted.

Prodrome: Within 24 hours preceding the headache, about 50 percent of migraineurs experience a prodrome, suggesting subtle disruptions of normal brain activity. These changes include alterations in mood (irritability, depression, euphoria, high or low energy levels) or sensory perception (overly sensitive to light, noise, touch, odors), food cravings (especially simple carbohydrates, like candy and cake), excessive yawning and speech or memory problems.

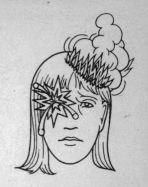

Aura: Within one hour preceding the headache, about 15 percent of migraineurs experience an aura, a discrete disruption of brain function. Usually visual, auras include flashing lights and shimmering zigzag lines encircling a central dark blind spot. At times, visual acuity diminishes, similar to the sensation of looking through a window splattered with rain. At times, there is numbness or the feeling of pins and needles around the lip or hand. Occasionally, auras may be profound, with loss of speech and vision or even hallucinations.

Headache: The headache of migraine is usually pulsating, occurs on only one side of the head and lasts 4 to 72 hours. Muscles in the neck and scalp may be tender. In addition, the person feels sick to the stomach and does not want to eat, move, see or hear. Going to bed in a dark, quiet room seems the best way to cope. Despite the usual pattern, migraine may occur on both sides of the head and alternate from side to side.

Resolution: The head pain subsides and the body regains normal homeostasis. The process may occur over several hours during sleep or rest, or the headache may end abruptly during vomiting or after an intense emotional experience.

Postdrome: After the head pain stops, most migraineurs experience a period lasting up to 24 hours when they feel drained, fatigued and tired. They are mentally dull and muscles ache. Emotions are frequently volatile, ranging from depression to euphoria.

Tension–type Headache

Tension–type headaches are common, accounting for nearly 90 percent of all headaches, and probably experienced by most people at some time during their lifetime. Frequently associated with fatigue and stress, these headaches generally respond to simple measures, such as rest or over-the-counter pain medicine. They occur 3 times more often in women than men and are commonly seen in family members. Yet tension headaches may become chronic, occurring 15 to 30 days a month, which often pushes the individual into seeking medical attention.

A tension–type headache is usually bilateral (pain on both sides of the head), consisting of a dull, steady ache.

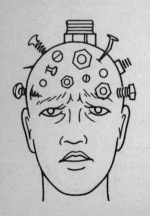

Muscle tenderness may accompany a tension headache as it does a migraine, but it is usually less severe. Factors that differentiate tension from migraine headaches include: 1) Disability is usually less, allowing individuals to continue to work with the headache; 2) Routine physical activity does not worsen the pain; 3) Nausea, vomiting and oversensitivity to lights and sounds do not generally accompany the headache; and 4) Tension–type headaches rarely awaken a person from sleep.

Mixed Headache

The mixed or tension-vascular headache shares features of both migraines and tension–type headaches. Usually, a baseline tension-like headache exists with attacks of migraine-like symptoms; it is as if a migraine is superimposed on a tension–type headache. Mixed headaches are frequently associated with analgesic overuse, depression, sleep disturbances and anxiety disorders.

Cluster Headache

Cluster headaches produce excruciating pain, affect men 6 times more frequently than women and afflict less than half a percent of individuals. The first attack strikes during the second or third decade of life. Those with cluster headaches are usually heavy smokers. Unlike migraines, cluster headaches do not appear in family members.

Individual headaches last 15 minutes to 3 hours, but these headaches "cluster," occurring up to several times a day for periods of 3 to 16 weeks. The headache may resolve for months to years and then strike again. Occasionally it becomes chronic. There appears to be seasonal variations, with spring or autumn often precipitating a cluster cycle.

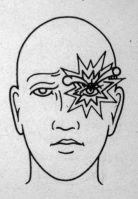

Cluster pain originates behind or around one eye and generally awakens the individual from sleep. The pain may radiate into the temple, jaw, nose, teeth or chin. The eyelids droop, the eyes tear. The face flushes and the nose congests. There is usually no nausea or vomiting. During an attack, the person is restless and agitated, pacing and desperate to find relief for the head pain. Alcohol, cold wind and heat blown into the face may initiate an attack during a cluster period.

Sinus Headache

A sinus headache is associated with inflammation of the sinus cavities, usually as a result of an infection or allergic reaction. The sinus headache is described as a deep, dull ache, located around the nose, sometimes extending into the forehead and ears. There is frequently a thick, purulent,

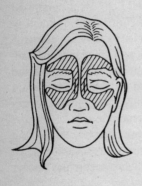

colored nasal discharge and a foul odor to the breath. At times the pain can become quite intense and disabling. This can last as long as the underlying condition exists. Over-the-counter medications often abolish the pain or relieve congestion. Lying down with a hot compress or humidifying the sinuses also curbs discomfort.

Rebound Headache

AN INDIVIDUAL WITH DAILY HEADACHES, WHO TAKES 100 ASPIRIN OR TYLENOL A MONTH, IS LIKELY EXPERIENCING A DRUG REBOUND HEADACHE.

A rebound headache occurs daily or almost daily, even though the individual frequently takes headache medication to counter the discomfort. Typically, the medication brings relief, but as it wears off, the headache returns. As the condition worsens, the medication becomes less effective. Eventually, the medications used to treat the headache perpetuate the headache cycle; going without medication results in a severe rebound headache. The drugs capable of producing rebound headache syndromes include over-the-counter analgesics (aspirin, Tylenol, Excedrin, Vanquish), caffeine, prescription pain medicines, sedatives and ergotamines.

> *"Something behind my left eye is about to explode. Even after the devastating pain stops, the time bomb keeps ticking."*

An estimated 2 percent of the general population suffers daily rebound headaches. The head pain often persists to varying degrees throughout the day, fluctuating in intensity from mild to moderately severe. The ache, usually diffuse or dull, is on both sides of the head, but at times may be localized to a specific area of the head. Symptoms characteristic of migraines may accompany the daily pain. An individual with daily headaches who takes 4–6 or more aspirin or acetaminophen (Tylenol) or much smaller quantities of prescription medications on a daily basis is likely experiencing drug rebound headaches.

The only effective treatment is to withdraw the person from the medication responsible for the rebound phenomena. Withdrawal symptoms are expected and need to be treated by a physician. The headache may intensify during the withdrawal process. Once the medication is out of the system, an alternative way to treat the headache will be prescribed.

Menstrual Migraine

The fluctuation of hormones, especially estrogen, during the menstrual cycle is associated with migraines in 60 percent of female migraineurs; 14 percent of them suffer migraines

The Stress of Headaches

I am 54 and have had a daily headache for the past 28 years. I graduated from engineering school and went through ranger training in the army without a headache. Not until I started my own business did my first headache strike. Some headaches were severe; most were mild. But I lived in constant fear of being struck down by a headache and not being able to function at my job. I discovered that Excedrin controlled my headaches. I took 2 to 8 tablets per day without fail. Excedrin became a permanent part of my life. About nine years ago, I had a grand mal seizure. I entered a pain and stress clinic where an attempt was made to wean me off Excedrin, without success. After I left the clinic, I still had daily headaches, but the severe ones left for more than a year. I continued daily Excedrin because I knew that if I stopped, the severe headaches would return. I finally admitted, three years ago, that Excedrin had become an addiction. There were many stresses in my life that I had not dealt with. I knew they were part of my headaches, too. But I could no longer tell where the headache ended and the Excedrin began.

STABLE LEVELS OF ESTROGEN MAY BE MIGRAINE-PROTECTIVE.

only at the time of menses. The headache begins just prior to the start of menstruation. Estrogen does not directly cause a migraine; in fact, during pregnancy and other high estrogen states, migraines are less frequent. Instead, a rapid decrease in estrogen levels is most likely to be associated with migraines, suggesting that stable levels may be migraine-protective. Hormonal levels near menses sensitize the headache threshold to influences from the environment.

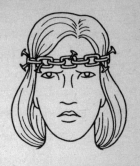

Menstrual migraines are generally more difficult to treat and last longer than other types of headaches. Once the menstrual susceptibility is discovered, a woman can compensate for other stressors and use medication to prevent or treat menstrual-related migraine.

Danger Signals

Only 1 out of 25,000 acute headaches is a symptom of a serious underlying disorder. The danger signals of headaches are:

1. The head pain is severe and new, unlike past headaches.
2. The head pain becomes worse over time.
3. The head pain begins with physical exertion, straining, coughing or sexual activity.
4. With the head pain, the person feels drowsy, confused, feverish or shows signs of physical decline.
5. The first headache occurs after the age of 40.

A physician needs to be consulted if any of the above symptoms appear.

WHAT TYPE OF HEADACHE DO I HAVE?

Yes *No*

____ ____ 1) Do you know what may be causing your headache? (Whiplash, diabetes, high blood pressure, eye strain)?

____ ____ 2) Has this type of headache occurred before?

____ ____ 3) Do you have more than one type of headache?

____ ____ 4) Does your neck, shoulder muscles or head junction feel tight and painful during the headache?

____ ____ 5) Is your headache pain dull and steady, like a constant pressure?

____ ____ 6) Does your headache feel like a tight band around your head?

____ ____ 7) Do you usually have one or more headaches per week?

____ ____ 8) Do your headaches usually begin later in the day?

____ ____ 9) Does your mother, father or any blood relative have similar headaches?

____ ____ 10) Does exertion (lifting, running, straining, sex) affect your headache?

____ ____ 11) Does nausea and/or vomiting occur during your headache?

____ ____ 12) Do you have any changes in vision (flashing lights, sensitivity to light, spots, blurred vision) before or during your headache?

____ ____ 13) Is your headache usually on one side of your head?

_____ _____ 14) Does your headache throb, pulsate or feel like it is pounding?

_____ _____ 15) Does your headache often awaken you in the early morning?

_____ _____ 16) (Females only) Is your headache associated with your menstrual cycle?

_____ _____ 17) Do moderate amounts of alcoholic beverages cause or aggravate your headache?

_____ _____ 18) Does chocolate, caffeine, cheese, milk, nuts, prepared meats, Oriental food or any other food cause or aggravate your headache?

_____ _____ 19) Does your headache last less than three hours?

_____ _____ 20) Does your headache occur daily for weeks at a time and then disappear for long periods?

_____ _____ 21) Do you have a watery red eye on the same side as the headache?

_____ _____ 22) Does your headache often awaken you shortly (1–3 hours) after falling asleep?

_____ _____ 23) Do you have any hearing problems, such as ringing, drainage or stuffiness in either ear?

_____ _____ 24) Do you have any facial pain, aching jaws, stuffiness or congestion along with your headache?

_____ _____ 25) Have you noticed any paralysis, muscle weakness, numbness, swallowing problems or speech changes during your headache?

_____ _____ 26) Has it been over 18 months since you visited a dentist?

_____ _____ 27) Have you had tests for headaches (X ray, CAT scan, MRI)?

___ ___ 28) Has your headache pattern changed in the last six months?

___ ___ 29) Do you take medication several times a week for your headache?

___ ___ 30) Do you experience a severe headache if you stop your headache medication?

Add the "Yes" responses. Score:

"Yes" responses to questions 4–9 indicate features of **tension headaches.**

"Yes" responses to questions 4 and 9–18 indicate features of **migraines.**

"Yes" responses to questions 13 and 19–22 indicate features of **cluster headaches.**

"Yes" responses to questions 24 and 26 in addition to other positive responses indicate features of **sinus headaches.**

"Yes" responses to questions 29 and 30 in addition to other positive responses indicate features of **rebound headaches.**

"Yes" responses to 3 and 25–28 or "No" responses to question 1 or 2 indicate the need to **see a physician.**

5

A NEW PARTNERSHIP: FINDING THE RIGHT DOCTOR

Within the medical system, the physician coordinates treatment, much as a symphony conductor organizes the sounds of an orchestra to produce a melody. As the diagnostician and prescriber of treatment, the doctor wields power. Finding the right physician is paramount to interrupting an established headache pattern.

Diagnosis

Proper treatment begins with a correct diagnosis. Yet surveys estimate that 60 percent of women and 70 percent of men with moderately to severely disabling headaches have not received a physician diagnosis. Most of these people have seen physicians, but for a variety of reasons, the headache problem was not adequately explored. Often, physicians do not screen patients for headaches or do not have the time to elicit a complete headache history. Patients and physi-

A PHYSICIAN CANNOT CURE HEADACHES, BUT HEADACHES CAN BE MANAGED.

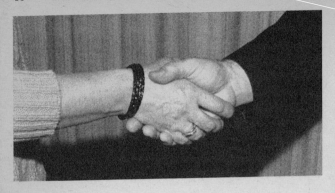

cians frequently interact only during an acute headache attack, ignoring the chronic nature of the disorder.

Compliance

When a headache sufferer seeks a cure from a physician,
there will always be disappointment. A physician cannot
cure headaches, but headaches can be managed. A partnership between the headache sufferer and the physician rests
on honesty and trust. The physician needs to hear how well
the prescribed treatment worked. Many migraineurs fear dis-
closing the truth to the physician because failed treatment
is often viewed as a failure of the patient. But a physician
willing to listen, to believe and to alter the medication to fit
your needs is a partner to help with your dilemma. Time is
needed to adjust medication to find relief. Be patient and
comply. Statistics reveal that one-half of headache sufferers
abandon their prescribed therapies, probably because they
become impatient with ineffective remedies. There are
other approaches. Many effective medications are available
and can be adjusted to fit individual needs. But unless the
physician receives accurate feedback about treatment, little
can be done.

Growing Up with Migraines

I grew up with migraines. My mother and father both had migraines. They would suffer in bed for days. The house was dark and dead still. Nothing helped. Mom saw one doctor, but the medicine affected her whole body, making things worse. She decided that the medication made her as sick as the headache. She never went back to the doctor.

I wasn't surprised when, at 13, I suffered my first migraine. I was afraid of them even though they struck only once in awhile. I had nightmares about their taking over my life like they did my parents'. I wanted to go to a doctor, but my father said there wasn't anything anyone could do. Every month, I took my turn lying in my bedroom with the shades pulled, an ice pack on my head, praying for the pain to end. The ritual was like a price I had to pay for being part of the family.

After I married, my headaches became more frequent. I used a lot of over-the-counter pain medication. At first, my husband felt sorry for me, but before long, he was frustrated by my headaches. I couldn't blame him. We'd plan something fun, but the boom would fall and I'd get a headache. Eventually I took medication all the time, hoping that it would prevent my headache from starting. Instead, the headaches got worse.

Finally, I went to my doctor. He referred me to a headache specialist. I didn't know doctors specialized in headaches. She understood my headache problem. She was easy to talk to and I liked her right away. She asked me to keep a diary. By recording my habits, I discovered that my diet and lifestyle were encouraging headaches. She taught me how to use my medication properly. The biggest plus was that her prescribed treatment worked.

Migraines are still with me, but not as often. I manage the headaches. I like being their manager instead of their victim. My husband and family finally understand this problem and are less critical. I wish Mom and Dad would have gotten help.

What Is Headache Disability?

Headache disability encompasses the activities that the individual cannot engage in due to pain, nausea, vomiting or other symptoms. Headache sufferers function at a level less than their potential. As a result, families, jobs, churches, teams and friends lose out. Migraineurs often find themselves becoming less social, saving their energy for work and insulating themselves from many outside influences that may initiate a migraine. Over a period of years, headache sufferers may lose promotions, friends, invitations, the promise of a better future and respect from their peers. A severely disabling headache totally incapacitates the person, usually requiring bed rest and forcing withdrawal from daily life. A moderately disabling headache causes the individual to restrict activities to those that are essential. A mildly disabling headache lowers efficiency, but

HEADACHE SUFFERERS FUNCTION AT A LEVEL LESS THAN THEIR POTENTIAL.

generally allows one to continue functioning at work and home.

Why People Do Not Seek Medical Treatment for Headaches

FAMILY

Many migraineurs have grown up in families where at least one other person suffered headaches. "Sick headaches" are a fact of life. The plan to beat the headache is for the person to withdraw from activities, seek solace in a dark, quiet room and take whatever medication is in the medicine cabinet. Headaches, to these people, are an affliction, accepted and suffered through because there is no known alternative. But what may have been true years ago is no longer valid today. Nearly all disabling headaches improve with proper treatment.

SEVERITY

People dread having their head pain complaints minimized. "It's only a headache" is every migraineur's fear when seeking professional help. "Is my headache bad enough to ask for help" is the question being weighed before a person submits himself to the humiliation of the emergency room or to making an appointment to see a physician. "It's just part of your PMS (Premenstrual Syndrome)" and "nobody dies of a headache" are phrases used to discount headaches. Won't a doctor say the same?

Headache sufferers themselves may attempt to down-play their pain, considering it a result of wrong living rather than an actual medical disorder. When

"I've burned out three neurologists."

The Path to Hope

I was 19 when I first went to a doctor about my headaches. The doctor seemed more interested in my starting birth control pills than in treating my headaches, even though I was not sexually active. He told me that I had migraines and I had to learn to live with them. He recommended aspirin, which I knew would not touch my headache. My headaches became worse. I was afraid that something was seriously wrong. I made an appointment with a neurologist who ordered all kinds of tests. Everything was fine, but he gave me a prescription and told me to come back if the medicine didn't work. Months later, I finally returned. He suggested medicine to prevent the attacks. I gained 25 pounds, but my headaches continued. I quit the medication. Since then, I've seen many more doctors, tried different medications and had more normal tests. Until now, I never thought I should be a part of my treatment. I've kept a diary and learned about the events that can contribute to my headaches. It's so simple and it's given me hope.

there are no flashing lights or vomiting, headaches may be attributed to something else, such as sinus infection. Frequently, only headaches that are really bad or associated with an aura are considered worthy of medical treatment. In short, headaches cover a wide range of symptoms and inadequate or improper treatment can increase headache frequency and prolong disability.

DEFEAT

Consulting a physician for a headache is admitting defeat, giving in to the head pain. Having to ask for professional help is focusing on the seriousness of the disorder. "Are headaches worth a visit to a doctor?" "Most people have headaches once in awhile and they don't go to the doctor." "There must be something wrong with me."

EXPENSE

Before seeking medical assistance, headache sufferers often weigh the cost against the anticipated benefit; "Seeing the doctor is expensive and probably won't help." In reality, though, suffering is more expensive than obtaining medical care. Migraines produce moderate to severe disability in 1 out of 11 adults. At times, they remain on the job with a migraine, reducing efficiency and increasing frustration. Over time, these factors may result in lost wages, missed promotions and disruption in a sense of well-being. Over a lifetime, such interference amounts to a loss of significant income. Estimates of lost productivity due to disabling headaches range from $7,000 per year for men and $4,000 per year for women.

Medical Barriers

Several medical barriers exist which deny proper medical treatment to those afflicted with headaches. Headaches have been a step-child of medicine. In medical training, the importance of headaches is often viewed as a symptom of a serious underlying disease, such as a brain tumor. Physicians are quick to exclude this rare possibility, attacking the headache symptom with a barrage of medical tests. When the tests fail to show underlying disease, they report the "good news," but fail to adequately address the headache itself.

HEADACHES HAVE NO TESTS TO DIAGNOSE THEIR PRESENCE.

Another problem is that headache disorders have no tests that can diagnose their presence. The diagnosis of headaches is largely made by a careful medical history. In the age of modern medicine, where technology reigns, headaches are an enigma. Physicians are often unwilling to invest the time necessary to understand the impact or seriousness of headaches and tend to minimize their importance. After all, no one ever dies from a migraine.

Finally, medical research has only recently validated a clear biologic basis for headaches and their treatment. Headache treatment in the past has largely focused on acute headache symptoms, such as pain or nausea. Unrestricted use of medicine for pain and other symptoms concerns physicians, who fear that overuse can lead to medical complications, such as addiction. As a result, physicians are reluctant to engage the headache patient in adequate therapy, predicting that treatment will be a never-ending cycle of prescription writing.

Finding the Balance

Many physicians take an interest in headache management, demonstrating the value of medical care for the control of headaches and the reduction of disability. There needs to be a partnership between patients and physicians where patients are afforded the opportunity to participate in management of their disorder. Because headaches are a chronic condition, the management style needs to be comprehensive, emphasizing education and self-monitoring.

Choosing a Physician

In choosing a physician, examine your own expectations and needs. Physicians may be educators and facilitators for those motivated to manage their headaches or prescription writers for those demanding an immediate "cure." Physicians can give guidelines for exploring the complex nature of an individual's headache problem, but cannot furnish all the answers. Physicians can prescribe medications as a valuable component of a headache program and teach the safe and proper use of these medications. They can be supportive during the trial-and-error of formulating a management program. Physicians can accurately diagnose headache problems and suggest headache specialists or psychologists to assist with complicated headache problems. Approaching a physician with realistic expectations of what is needed, and possible, will enhance the relationship for both physician and patient.

PRIMARY CARE PHYSICIANS

Your family doctor can diagnose and manage most headaches. Share your assessment of the headache problem with the physician. List the symptoms you experience and the impact they have on your life. Share the results of treatments you have tried. During the interview, notice the physician's level of interest in your problem. Assess if this is a physician willing to understand you as well as your headache.

Primary physicians, such as family doctors, internists, pediatricians and obstetricians/gynecologists, see the majority of the headache population. Complicated cases may call for special diagnostic considerations and consultation with other specialists. Primary care physicians coordinate these consultations while managing patients' medical needs. Specialists, like family physicians and internists, are accustomed to helping people manage chronic conditions. As headaches continue to be more fully understood, medical care will improve.

PHYSICIAN REFERRAL

PHYSICIAN REFERRAL

If you do not have a physician or the physician you met did not seem responsive to your specific needs, seek another doctor from a local medical society. In addition, members of a headache support group comprise a valuable information resource for firsthand experiences with different physicians. By asking knowledgeable people for suggestions, you will find physicians who understand and enjoy managing headaches.

Treatment Plan

A treatment plan is a set of suggestions for managing your headaches. More than a prescription, a treatment plan begins with an understandable explanation of the diagnosis. Included is a review of the components of your headaches and ways to improve your health, such as through changes in lifestyle, diet, exercise and by relieving stress. How and when to take medication may be a significant part of the plan. Follow-up plans are essential.

Initial Visit

When making an appointment with a physician, be prepared. Review your diary and write down what you have learned about your headache pattern. Pay special attention to foods, the weather, stress and, for women, association with menstruation. Know your headache symptoms and organize them to help you convey them to your doctor. Send results of tests and medical records to the doctor before your visit. Write down all medications you use for headaches, especially over-the-counter products. Know your insurance coverage. Many companies exclude or pay less for important therapies, such as biofeedback. Others have confusing clauses about pre-existing conditions or exclude certain medications. If you have doubts, ask a representative of the insurance company for an explanation.

A complete medical evaluation may require more than one visit. In addition, follow-up visits to review treatment response are essential. Ask for educational materials for a better understanding of the treatment plan. A well-organized visit to the doctor will likely be satisfying and enlightening.

After your visit with the physician, use the diary to evaluate the effectiveness of treatment and record any problems you may experience with medication. This record will be invaluable for refining treatment in the future. If you have significant difficulties before the scheduled follow-up appointment, report them to your physician.

Headache Specialists

Headache specialists are health professionals with a declared interest in headaches who direct much of their clinical practice toward treating and studying headache patients. Most commonly, they are neurologists, internists, family physicians, psychiatrists or psychologists. Their expertise and familiarity with headache problems assist individuals who are suffering from complicated headache problems. Several professional organizations are devoted to the study of headaches and most headache specialists belong to one or more of these groups.

Headache Clinics

Most areas of the country have a headache specialty clinic nearby. These clinics generally offer a comprehensive approach to difficult headache problems, providing coordinated professional services from several different disciplines. In this way, the headache patient is evaluated from various perspectives and a comprehensive treatment plan is created.

Past treatment, medication and medical testing are reviewed. Patterns of medication use, adequacy of coping strategies and family dynamics are also assessed. Diet, posture and lifestyle are analyzed. From this comprehensive assessment, a treatment plan is constructed.

A multi-disciplinary approach relies on the expertise of physicians, psychologists, physical therapists and nurses. Physicians usually coordinate the treatment program, ensuring accuracy of diagnosis and directing medication adjustments. Psychologists assess the impact of psychological factors, such as depression, anxiety and family dynamics, on headache symptomatology. They direct biofeedback training and teach the patient and family effective coping skills. Nutritionists or specially trained nurses examine diet and lifestyle factors that possibly contribute to complicated headache problems. Physical therapists evaluate and treat structural and postural problems, and demonstrate to families and patients techniques to maintain physical comfort and relieve tension. Difficult headache syndromes occasionally require hospitalization or intense outpatient therapy. Programs may require individuals to participate in headache therapy for several hours each day. These intense programs generally last 2 to 3 weeks and immerse the headache sufferer in treatment.

MEDICAL VISIT WORKSHEET

Preparation before the visit:

1) Keep an accurate daily diary at least one month before you visit the doctor.

2) Review the diary record. Pinpoint the factors that seem important to your headache pattern (see "Headache Diary," Chapter 3).

3) Separate different headache types.
    Tension
    Migraine
    Sinus
    Other

4) Record the symptoms associated with your headache.
    Prodrome
    Aura (if present)
    Headache:
        Location
        Quality of pain
        Associated symptoms:
            Nausea/vomiting
            Sensitivity to light/sound
            Muscle tenderness
            Relationship to activity
        Duration
        Treatment:
            Past
            Present
            Effectiveness
            Side effects
        Disability

5) Postdrome (how you feel after the headache).

6) Previous evaluations.
    Medical evaluations
    Psychology and biofeedback experience
    Tests (X rays, CAT scans, MRIs, EEGs) and results

7) Other health problems.

8) Medications, including over-the-counter, herbs and vitamins.

Visiting the physician:

1) Bring a concise report of your headache pattern.

2) Ask questions about your headaches.

3) Be honest about symptoms, treatment attempts and concerns.

4) Explain your expectations.

5) Explore other management options.
   Biofeedback
   Physical therapy
   Smoking cessation
   Lifestyle modifications
   Headache support groups

6) Establish management goals.

7) Ask for printed information about headaches and medications.

8) Understand how and when to use your medication.

9) Schedule follow-up visits.

After the physician visit:

1) Reorganize your treatment program.
   Create the headache-protective environment
   Investigate and eliminate headache "triggers"
   Preventative headache medications
   Acute treatment strategy
      First-line treatment
      Second-line treatment

2) Continue your diary record.

3) Chart responses to medication.
   Effectiveness
   Side effects

4) Contact your physician's office with significant problems.

5) Comply with recommendations.

6) Keep follow-up appointments.

6

DIET, ENVIRONMENT AND HEADACHES

Diet

The human body processes food into usable nutrients and waste products. Every cell in our body is replaced many times during a lifetime. The materials for this renewal process come from our diet. We are what we eat.

Over millions of years, nature has perfected the digestive system. But the modern American diet has changed radically over the last 40 years. Food comes from all corners of the globe. To preserve freshness, man-made chemicals are added; trace amounts of herbicides, pesticides and fertilizers are standard ingredients of the daily diet. How these chemicals affect our health is unknown, but dietary factors seem to account, at least in part, for the 60 percent increase in migraine prevalence over the last decade.

Certain dietary factors predictably trigger headaches. Many foods and chemicals assault the system, leading to headaches or other illnesses, like cancer or heart disease. There is little doubt that diet is an important part of human health. Becoming aware of what we eat and making conscientious choices about what we put into our bodies can enhance health and may decrease headache frequency.

Eliminating Dietary Triggers

Solving the mystery of dietary contributions to headaches takes work; first, to discover the chemicals that precipitate headaches and, second, to identify the foods that contain these chemicals. To complicate the process, certain foods may trigger a headache occasionally but not 100 percent of the time. Instead, a dietary trigger may add to the vulnerability of the nervous system by increasing the overall stress load. A small amount of a certain chemical may be tolerated when other stressors are minimal. But when a larger amount is consumed or there are other headache precipitants present, headaches strike.

A major problem is knowing the foods that hide headache-producing chemicals. Monosodium glutamate (MSG), for example, is a chemical known to trigger headaches in many people. Yet it is described by different terms in various foods, such as *hydrogenated vegetable protein*, *natural preservatives* or simply *seasonings*. Often, the more one is aware of what to avoid, the more confusing it is to know what one is eating.

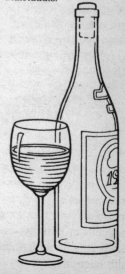

Red wine contains alcohol and tyramine, both of which may provoke headaches in sensitive individuals.

Learning About Diet

To understand the relationship between diet and headache, begin with the Headache Diary and read labels on food. In the kitchen, hang up a list of foods and chemicals that can cause headaches. Whenever a headache occurs, review the Diary for chemical factors that may have contributed. Even though an identified factor may not be implicated with every headache, after several attacks are analyzed, a pattern may emerge.

DIETARY FACTORS IN MIGRAINES	SUBSTITUTES
· Alcohol, red wine, champagne, beer	· White wine, clear liquor, non-alcoholic beverages
· Aged cheese: sharp cheddar, Swiss, provolone	· Cottage cheese, ricotta
· Citrus fruits	· Other fruits
· Aged, cured or processed meats: hot dogs, lunch meats, bacon	· Freshly prepared meat/fish
· Sour cream	· Yogurt (not homemade)
· Pickled, fermented or marinated foods: herring, sardines, anchovies, capers	· Freshly prepared fish
· Food additives: meat tenderizers, MSG, soy sauce	· Natural spices
· Peanuts, peanut butter	· Almond butter
· Homemade yeast breads and yogurt	· Breads/food without active yeast cultures
· Chocolate	· Carob
· Caffeine-containing beverages: colas, teas, coffee	· Herbal teas, fruit juices (bottled or fresh, but not citrus), water
· Nutrasweet	· Honey

Specific Dietary Factors

Many dietary chemicals provoke migraines by interfering with normal regulation of blood vessels or the nervous system. Because migraineurs are susceptible to this action, an elimination of these chemicals can reduce attacks.

Food or chemical sensitivities are highly individual, making a complete list of these chemicals impractical if not impossible. But, the foods commonly identified to provoke headaches are included on the list on page 62.

ALCOHOL

Alcohol often provokes headaches. In excess, alcohol can cause a hangover headache, a toxic process different from the triggering mechanism in other types of headaches. For those with active cluster headaches or migraines, even small quantities of alcohol can precipitate a headache. Alcohol dilates—or opens up—blood vessels, causing flushed cheeks and red eyes. This stretching of blood vessels may provoke headache attacks during a period of vulnerability.

Certain types of alcohol are more likely to trigger headaches than others. Red wine, for instance, is a potent trigger for migraines. White wine and clear liquors are the best-tolerated forms of alcohol for migraineurs. But, even these can precipitate a migraine when other headache-producing factors are present.

NITRATES AND NITRITES

Nitrates and nitrites are preservatives found in prepared meats like hot dogs, sausage and bacon. Also used to preserve meat at grocery stores and salads in restaurants, these chemicals dilate and stretch blood vessels, often leading to a migraine in a susceptible individual.

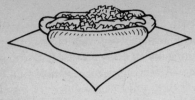

The preservatives in a hot dog may precipitate a migraine in a susceptible person.

TYRAMINE

Tyramine is an amino acid that is an essential building block for the body. Used by the body to make adrenaline and other necessary substances, tyramine constricts blood vessels and, in the process, may produce headaches. Tyramine is found in high concentrations in red wine, beer and aged cheeses. It must be avoided while on medications called monoamine oxidase (MAO) inhibitors as the interaction between these drugs and tyramine can produce dangerous elevations in blood pressure. MAO inhibitors are prescribed by physicians to treat high blood pressure, depression or, at times, migraines. Consult your doctor or pharmacist if you have any questions about this class of medications.

FOODS CONTAINING NITRATES

Bacon	Liverwurst
Bratwurst	Pastrami
Beef jerky	Pork and beans
Corn dogs	Salami
Corned beef	Sausage
Ham	Smoked fish
Hot dogs	Spam
Lunch meats	Turkey lunch meats

CAFFEINE

Caffeine interferes with headache management through several different means and its contribution to headaches is often underestimated. Caffeine constricts blood vessels and, in sufficient quantities, can result in a headache. More commonly, though, daily use of caffeine (more than 2 cups of coffee or 2 cans of soda pop) causes the nervous system to rely on caffeine. If caffeine is suddenly withdrawn, a headache can result.

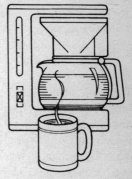

The weekend migraine, for example, strikes after a work-week of coffee that maintains high levels of caffeine. During the weekend, caffeine consumption is decreased, resulting in a headache that is often relieved by coffee or other caffeinated beverages. Caffeine-withdrawal headaches also commonly occur in the early morning, after a caffeine-free night.

As a stimulant, caffeine interferes with sleep, which may produce an ineffective sleep pattern. Without proper sleep, the system becomes easily overstressed, setting the stage for a headache cycle. Because caffeine blocks the normal breakdown of adrenaline, a potent stimulant of the nervous system, the body is maintained in a state of alert.

Caffeine or similar chemicals are found in coffee, some teas, many sodas and chocolate. In addition, several over-the-counter pain medications and sinus preparations contain caffeine. Eliminating or at least minimizing caffeine usually lessens headaches. To avoid a withdrawal headache, slowly decrease caffeine over a two-week period. Because decaffeinated coffee may contain other caffeine-like chemicals, coffee may have to be eliminated from the diet to stop the influence of caffeine as a headache trigger.

CAFFEINE CONTENT OF
SELECTED FOODS AND DRUGS

Coffee (5 oz.)	*Average in milligrams (mg.)*
Drip	137
Instant	60

Teas (6 oz.)	
American, black	46
Imported, black	32
Mint	50
Oolong	40

Soft drinks (12 oz.)	
Coca-Cola	45
Diet Coke	45
Dr Pepper	40
Ginger ale	0
Grape soda	0
Mountain Dew	54
Orange soda	0
Pepsi-Cola	38
Diet Pepsi	36
Root beer	0 (not all brands)
Seven-Up	0
Sparkling water	0
Sprite	0

Chocolate (1 oz.)	
Sweet (dark) chocolate	20
Hershey	23

Nonprescription drugs (1 pill)	
Excedrin	130
Midol	64
No Doz	200
Vanquish	66
Anacin	64
Dexatrim	200

Prescription drugs (1 pill)

Cafergot capsule	100
Darvon compound	32
Fiorinal tablet	40

MONOSODIUM GLUTAMATE (MSG)

Monosodium glutamate is a popular additive and seasoning found in many foods. Often listed on food labels as *hydrolyzed vegetable protein, natural food additives* or *seasonings,* MSG appears in a variety of food products, from canned and instant soups to Oriental dishes. By constricting blood vessels, MSG may initiate migraines in susceptible individuals.

FOODS CONTAINING MSG

Accent seasoning	Frozen pizza
Bacon bits	Gelatins
Baking mixes	Oriental food
Bouillon cubes	Potato chips
Bread stuffing	Pot pies
Breaded foods	Processed cheeses
Canned meats	Processed meats
Cheese dips	Relishes
Clam chowder	Salad dressings
Corn chips	Salt substitutes
Croutons	Seasonings
Dry roasted peanuts	Soups
Frozen dinners	Soy sauce

CITRUS FRUIT

A group of chemicals commonly found in citrus fruits, such as grapefruit, oranges, lemons and limes, may produce headache attacks. These chemicals act like certain messenger chemicals in the nervous system and interfere with the headache-protective balance. Not all headache sufferers are susceptible to these chemicals, but they may be a precipitant.

CHOCOLATE

Theobromides are chemicals found in chocolate that can provoke migraines. Chocolate also contains caffeine, which may intensify the headache-producing effects of theobromides. Migraine prodromes frequently include craving carbohydrates like chocolate, which can make its association as a migraine precipitant more difficult to assess.

Positive Dietary Factors

Tryptophan: Tryptophan, an amino acid, is the building block of serotonin, the neurochemical that enhances sleep, relaxation, a calm mood and protects against headaches. Obtainable in health food stores as a dietary supplement, tryptophan was used to counteract insomnia and a general sense of nervousness. But in 1990, the Federal Drug Administration (FDA) prohibited the sale of tryptophan because a contaminated batch entered the United States and caused a rare form of muscle disease in a few people. Even though many experts recognize that tryptophan itself was not responsible for this reaction, the FDA has not lifted its ban. Despite its unavailability as a food supplement, tryptophan occurs naturally in milk, poultry, wild game, legumes and cottage cheese. By eating these foods at least 4 or 5 times a week, an adequate supply of tryptophan may be maintained in the body.

Omega-3-Fatty Acids: Omega-3-fatty acids are a type of fat found in oily fish, such as cod, salmon and sardines. Available as a food supplement, Omega-3-fatty acids in doses of 16 grams per day reduce the frequency of migraine attacks in many people.

Vitamins: Vitamins are important dietary chemicals that assist many chemical reactions in the body and are necessary for health. Considerable controversy exists over the amount of vitamins that are necessary for optimal health. Several studies, however, suggest that quantities greater than the Minimum Daily Requirements (MDR) protect health.

Elimination Diet

Day 1   Eat your normal diet.

Day 2   Eliminate chemicals from diet, such as food additives, over-the-counter drugs, nicotine, alcohol, caffeine.

Day 3   Begin diet of brown rice, fresh or boiled fruit (not citrus) and vegetables, noncaffeinated herbal teas, and 8 glasses of water per day. Continue for 10 days.

Day 13   Add one type of food and test the body's response. Add bread, fruit or dairy products. Eat a moderate amount, such as 3–4 slices of bread, 4 oz. of cheese or 8 oz. of milk.

Day 17   Add meat, only one kind per day.

Day 18   You may choose to add processed foods one at a time to test the body's reaction.

Day 19   If the body acts negatively with headache, nausea, stomach upset or intestinal problems, avoid that substance for two weeks. Retest and, if the same reaction occurs, eliminate that substance from your diet.

A recent study showed that people supplementing their diet with additional vitamin C lived an average of 6 years longer than those who did not. Likewise, beta carotene and other free-radical scavengers (vitamin C and vitamin E) exhibit health benefits when taken as supplements. Under stress, unstable molecules increase and have the potential to harm body cells. Antioxidants (beta carotene and vitamins C and E) defuse these unstable molecules and help protect the body. Even though firm statements about dietary supplements are not possible at present, research suggests that vitamins may play a role in headache protection. Common sense dictates that by providing the body with health sustaining supplements, the entire system benefits. Discuss the issue of vitamins and food supplements with your physician and research their proper use.

Food Allergies

The scientific support of food allergies as a significant influence on headaches is controversial. But, on a practical level, headache sufferers often recognize that eating certain foods results in a headache. The mechanism of food allergies is complicated. The food substance initiates an immune response that mobilizes the entire system, increases stress and paves the way for headaches.

Generally, individuals susceptible to headaches from food are allergic to many other things in the environment. Almost any food is capable of being an allergen, but dairy products are very common sources. In susceptible people, the proteins in milk trigger an immune response, producing symptoms such as nasal congestion, sneezing, bloating, diarrhea, constipation or chronic headaches. Elimination of milk products or other food allergens for several weeks can ease the symptoms and enhance physical well-being. Skin tests and desensitization shots are promoted by some, but are not widely accepted. The only way to adequately test if food allergies play a part in one's headache syndrome is to go on an elimination diet. Eggs, milk, wheat, citrus and corn are the most common food allergies.

The Elimination Diet

Devoid of most known allergens, the elimination diet is also a process of removing food additives, preservatives, nicotine, alcohol and caffeine from the daily menu. The individual eats foods that are gentle on the immune system, such as brown rice, fruit (not citrus) and vegetables. Noncaffeinated herbal teas, unprocessed fruit and vegetable juice and at least 8 glasses of water per day are encouraged.

An elimination diet removes potentially toxic chemicals from the system. Headaches may actually increase during the first few days of this diet. If, however, headache symptoms then resolve or dramatically improve, food sensitivities may be an important contributor to the headache pattern. If that is the case, the diet is slowly expanded and the body's response to the addition of certain foods is carefully gauged. If a headache returns after eating specific foods, they are eliminated from the diet.

Elimination diets are not necessary for everyone with headaches. Chronic, frequent headaches that have not responded well to treatment and lifestyle adjustments may respond to elimination diets. Eating a healthy diet, however, makes everyone feel better.

Environment

The body is constantly adjusting to changes in the environment. Many atmospheric conditions may precipitate headaches. Pollutants in the air or water may create metabolic stress. The challenge lies in identifying the culprits that are capable of producing headaches.

Carbon Monoxide: Exposure to carbon monoxide, even small amounts, can cause headaches. Many migraineurs are highly sensitive to the effects of carbon monoxide on the blood vessels. Carbon monoxide is a byproduct of cigarette smoking. Statistically, smokers have a higher incidence of migraines and their migraines are more resistant to treatment if they continue to smoke. Secondhand smoke also causes headaches. Less frequently, carbon monoxide escapes from faulty furnaces or automobile exhaust systems and produces headaches.

> *"When there is a drastic change in weather, the right side of my head becomes dull, like dead wood, and pulsates. My right eye wants to close, like it's giving up."*

Perfumes and Noxious Odors: Many migraineurs report the sudden onset of a migraine after exposure to certain odors and smells. Only a few molecules, a brief whiff of the wrong chemical, assaults the nervous system and mobilizes a full-fledged migraine attack. The odors most likely to launch this process are strong scents, such as perfumes, cleaning products or sprays.

Weather: Sudden changes in weather are a common headache precipitant. As storm fronts approach an area, changes in barometric pressure or in ionization of the air affect the headache sufferer, producing a migraine attack.

Other Environmental Factors: Changes in altitude that occur with flying or visiting the mountains or seashore, bright sunlight, fluorescent lighting and computer screens have all been designated as migraine precipitants.

ENVIRONMENTAL FACTORS WHICH CAN
PRECIPITATE HEADACHES

- Glaring lights
- Physical exertion
- Changes in weather
- High humidity
- Cold food or beverages
- Pungent odors
- Perfumes
- Fluorescent lights
- Computer screens
- Glasses or contact lenses that need adjustment

Identifying the body's response to the environment requires awareness and sensitivity. After suffering through several headache attacks and much trial-and-error, the answers begin to emerge.

Insights gained from the Headache Diary are invaluable. Even though many situational factors can be controlled, some cannot. The goal is to create the most healthy, restorative environment possible. Simple measures, such as healthy diet, clean smoke-free air, health-enhancing behaviors and avoiding specific chemical and physical triggers, minimize headache frequency.

> THE GOAL IS TO CREATE THE MOST HEALTHY, RESTORATIVE ENVIRONMENT POSSIBLE.

7

EXERCISE

The body is an organ of expression. Exercise is necessary to interact with the environment. When the body is ill, it shuts down to conserve energy and heal itself. At times, headache sufferers continue to go on despite the pain. This desensitizes communication between the mind and the body; the mind is ignoring the body's plea for rest. Regular exercise is one way to re-establish a healthy interchange between mind and body.

Listen to the body to discover the right amount of exercise. Too much or too little may precipitate a headache, especially if it is a change from normal activity levels. Exercise improves body mechanics, reduces the wear-and-tear of stress, conditions the body and creates body awareness. Choose a type of exercise that is fun, exhilarating and can be repeated often, at least 3 times a week. In the long run, frequent exercise increases health and boosts the threshold for avoiding headaches.

Body Mechanics

Muscles support and move the body through space. Usually paired, muscle groups counterbalance each other. As one muscle contracts, another stretches. As long as these groups of muscles work in concert, the support system provides locomotion.

Muscles are divided into two interrelated systems. Static muscles are used primarily for posture, and phasic muscles generate strength and activity.

STATIC MUSCLES/POSTURE

The muscles for posture (static muscles) hold the body in space and oppose the effects of gravity. Small muscles grouped along the neck, spine, shoulder girdle and pelvis form the major static muscle groups. These unique muscles are able to contract over long periods of time without fatigue.

Static muscles are more prone to injury and overuse than phasic muscles. When static muscles become overfatigued, phasic muscles take over to uphold posture. Phasic muscles are ill-suited for the workload and postural imbalances often result, producing pain and stiffness in the neck, shoulders, back or pelvis.

PHASIC MUSCLES/STRENGTH

Phasic muscles, like the biceps, triceps and quadriceps, are designed for strength. Phasic muscles generate power quickly, but cannot sustain contraction over long periods of time.

Most exercise programs focus on the phasic muscle mass and assume that postural muscles are strong enough to support and maintain correct posture during exercise activity. For someone in good physical condition at the start of an exercise program, this is probably true. But, for many, pos-

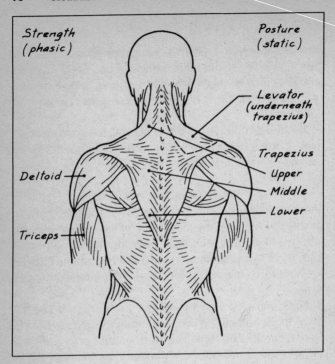

Muscles

ture needs to be improved prior to phasic muscle exercise. Otherwise, injury may result.

Muscle Mechanics and Headaches

Frequent bouts of head pain can result in chronic fatigue of muscles, especially in the head, neck and shoulders. To prevent head movement during a headache, the shoulder muscles draw up and the neck tightens, much like a turtle receding into its shell. The phasic muscles attempt to rescue the fatigued postural muscles, but these, too, tire quickly and normal muscle mechanics are disrupted.

During prolonged muscle contraction, blood flow to the muscle is reduced by the increased muscle tension compressing the blood vessels. This means that there is reduced oxygen available for the muscle to use. Nature considered this need and provided muscle tissue with mechanisms of maintaining contractions under conditions

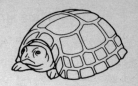

Stress draws up the muscles of the shoulders and tightens the neck, much like a turtle receding into its shell.

of reduced oxygen. When this occurs, however, the muscles are unable to burn sugar efficiently. Instead of sugar breaking down into carbon dioxide, which can readily be evacuated from the tissue, sugar breaks down into lactic acid. Removal of lactic acid from the tissue is a more difficult process. Nature's plan for lactic acid is to have it metabolized into carbon dioxide once the muscle is relaxed and blood flow is re-established.

During a headache, muscle tissue may be unable to replenish oxygen and lactic acid builds up. This irritates the muscle, resulting in pain and further muscle contraction. If the muscle is not relaxed, the muscle becomes irritable and prone to injury. Even between headaches, tender spots remain in the muscles of the neck and shoulders.

As these tender spots become areas of chronic muscle contraction, they pull on nerves and support structures in the surrounding area. This can produce pain and further muscle spasms. When pain spreads to areas outside of the muscle itself, the tender points are called *trigger points*. The nerve input from these areas increases the vulnerability of the headache threshold and propagates headaches.

Building an Exercise Program

An adequate exercise program consists of five phases.
1) Increase body awareness and breathing mechanics that establish a basis for exercise.
2) Apply this awareness to the sitting posture.
3) Transfer correct posture into the standing position.
4) Move these mechanics into daily activity.
5) Establish an aerobic exercise program. Exercise programs that begin with the basics help establish proper muscle balance.

Phase 1: Exercise for Body Awareness

Excessive muscle tension signals the approach of fatigue. By readjusting the postural dynamics before the muscles reach the point of spasm, muscle irritability can be avoided.

Exercises to increase awareness of muscle balance are simple to learn, but complex to master.

BODY AWARENESS EXERCISE

Lie on a firm, but comfortable surface, such as a carpeted floor. Place a 1 or 2 inch soft-covered book under the back of the head and drop the chin slightly to relax the muscles in the back of the neck. To position the head correctly, tip the chin gently downward. Place the hands on the lower abdomen and bend the knees, keeping the feet flat on the floor 12–18 inches apart. Place a soft towel under each elbow for support. Gently cough; use your hands to feel the muscles in the abdomen that moved during the cough. Breathe deeply from these muscles in the lower abdomen.

While breathing deeply and slowly, notice the position of your body. Adjust the chin and muscles in the back of

Abdominal Breathing

Abdominal breathing may feel awkward at first because many people are in the habit of taking quick, shallow breaths from the upper chest. Breathing from the abdomen creates an ideal oxygen exchange in the lungs and induces the body to relax. Practice this type of breathing until it becomes automatic.

the neck until they feel comfortable. If the shoulders are rolled forward and lifted off the floor, relax them. With each breath, allow gravity to move them gently downward. If this seems difficult, a small towel rolled and placed along the spine of the upper back will assist the proper positioning.

Concentrate on the chest and the air moving in and out of the lungs. Is breathing smooth and effortless? Feel the breath filling the lungs. Focus on your lower back and pelvis. Are the back and pelvis comfortably stretched out? If not, with each breath, relax the muscles and allow the spine to lengthen. Is the pelvis tight? Are the muscles of the legs contracted and restricting the pelvis? Breathe deeply and slowly until the tension releases.

Repeat this sequence until the body relaxes; the shoulders, spine and pelvis lie flat against the floor; and the lungs seem to breathe themselves. Practice this exercise for 10 minutes twice a day. During the exercise, focus attention on the muscles of the neck, spine and pelvis. With practice, awareness shifts from the head to inside the body, subtly changing postural muscles. After several weeks, balanced posture will feel natural. During the day's activities, there will be a greater awareness of muscles about to fatigue. This information motivates you to adjust behavior to refresh the body rather than exhaust it. This awareness helps you find a comfortable posture for biofeedback or sleep.

Phase 2: Moving into the Sitting Posture

After the mechanics of Phase 1 have been mastered (usually 2 or 3 weeks of daily practice), move that feeling of balanced posture into a sitting position. Using a comfortable, but firm chair, sit in front of a mirror to observe your posture.

1) Do the feet rest comfortably on the floor?
2) Is the pelvis straight?
3) Is the back perpendicular to the pelvis?
4) Are the shoulders level?
5) Does the head look straight?

Move away from the backrest of the chair and adjust your position until it feels comfortable. With your eyes closed, breathe deeply and focus on areas of tension or discomfort. Move into balance by quieting pressure. As the body achieves a natural postural position, tightness drains from the body and is replaced with relaxed composure.

In this position, with the chin neutral or slightly tucked in, imagine the spine stretching. This exercises the static muscles and counteracts the effects of gravity. The sensation is much like feeling as if you are growing. Concentrate on using the spinal muscles instead of merely lifting the chin and head.

To avoid fatigue, practice initially for only a short period of time. Feel the developing fatigue and adjust your position into one that relieves the tired muscles. Repeat these exercises until you can maintain a comfortable balanced posture for at least 15 minutes without fatiguing.

Include this new awareness in your day-to-day activities. Frequently assess your posture when at your desk. Abdominal breathing initiates the relaxation response and promotes postural adjustment. A sense of comfort is the indicator of correct posture. Because one posture cannot be comfortable all the time, begin with a balanced posture and make corrections frequently throughout the day.

When sitting at a desk, be certain that your chair fits your frame with your feet resting flat against the floor. The working surface needs to be within easy reach, allowing you to bring your work close to your body. At least once an hour, assess muscle tension and readjust. Get up and walk around. Exercise at your desk to relax fatiguing muscles.

DESKSIDE EXERCISES

Exercise #1: Thumbing
Stand with your arms relaxed at your side. Inhale. Exhale and rotate your thumbs outward. The movement of the muscles of your shoulders, neck, arms and upper back dissolves an accumulation of tension. Repeat 3 to 5 times.

Exercise #2: Chinning
The head leads the rest of the body. The way the head sits on the body determines the alignment of the bones and muscles. To lighten the load of a head that is pressed by demands, regain the natural head position by inhaling and tucking in the chin. As you exhale, stick out your chin. The curve of the neck is exaggerated, releasing a buildup of uncompleted tasks. Do this 3 to 5 times. Finish with the erect position.

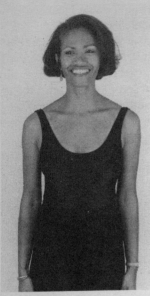

Stand with your arms relaxed at your sides and inhale.

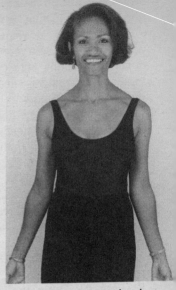

Exhale and rotate your thumbs outward, dissolving tension in the upper body.

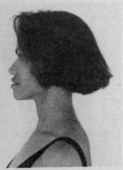

Regain the natural head position by inhaling and tucking in your chin.

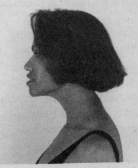

Exhale and stick out your chin, exaggerating the curve of the neck and releasing tension.

Exercise #3: Shouldering

As the muscles on top of the shoulders become tight, the shoulders are pulled. To soothe this strain, place a small rolled towel under each arm, making a fulcrum. Softly pat the palms of the hands toward the thighs, stroking life into the shoulders.

Exercise #4: Trapezing

The upper trapezius muscle attaches the shoulder blade to the back of the head. Often the upper trapezius is overused, producing an imbalance in the trapezius muscle group. When the muscles on the top of the shoulder blade are overdominant, they become shortened and stronger than the middle and lower trapezius, intended to counterbalance the upper trapezius. The upper overfunctions, while the lower and middle underfunction.

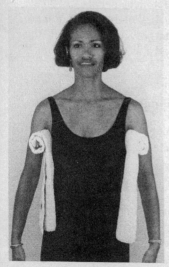

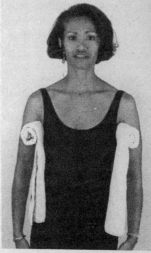

Place a small rolled towel under each arm.

Softly pat the palms of your hands toward the thighs, stroking life into the shoulders.

To relieve tension in the upper trapezius muscle, this exercise strengthens the middle and lower trapezius muscles, sharing the workload.

While standing, inhale and assume a neutral, natural posture with arms down at the sides. Inhale again. As you exhale, pinch the shoulder blades down and together. Inhale again, but as you exhale, press the shoulder blades down and together only one-half as far as the first time.

Exercise #5: Minishrugs

As a person becomes weighed down with problems, the overused trapezius muscles tire and the shoulders slump under the burden. Rest your arms at your side and relax the shoulders. As you inhale, elevate the shoulders as high as you can. Exhale and relax the shoulders. With the next breath, lift your shoulders only one-half as high as you did before. Exhale and relax the shoulders. Finally, as you inhale, raise the shoulders only one-half of the last lift. You are barely lifting your shoulders, but you are exercising the small postural muscles that need relief. Repeat the small movement exercise 3 to 5 times.

Phase 3: Standing Posture

Stand in front of a full-length mirror with your feet spread comfortably apart, about 18 inches or the width of your shoulders.

Observe your posture:

· Is your head squarely in the middle of the shoulders or is there a slight rotation of the head or shoulders?
· Is one shoulder higher or carried in front of the other?
· When you take a deep breath, does the chest expand fully or is the breath originating from the upper chest?
· Are the skin folds along your torso symmetrical?

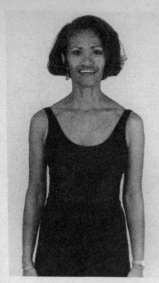 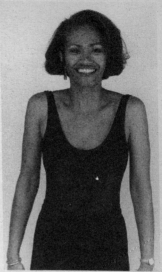

Rest your arms at your sides, relax the shoulders and exhale.

As you inhale, elevate the shoulders. With each shrug, lessen the elevation of the shoulders until they move only slightly. These minishrugs exercise the small postural muscles.

- Are the hip bones the same height?
- Are your feet comfortably balanced on the floor?

Turn to the side:
- Is your head directly over the shoulders or is it positioned out in front of the body?
- Is the chin in a neutral position?
- Are the shoulders sloped forward?
- Is the lower back straight or is there a swayback posture?
- Are you standing tall or do you slouch?

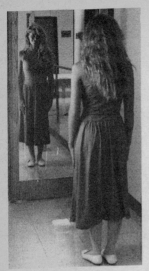
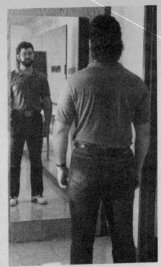

Observe your posture in a mirror.

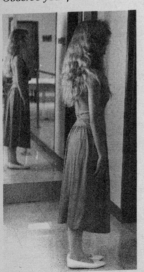
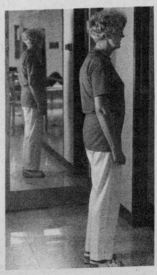

Turn to the side and assess your posture.

Finally, assess your posture from behind. This can be done by holding a second mirror or by having a friend assist you:

- Is the spine straight or is there a curvature?
- Is the pelvis square or is one dimple in the lower back higher than the other?
- Are the muscles of the buttocks relaxed or tense?
- Are the knees locked in full extension or positioned in a relaxed posture?
- Do you feel balanced?

Repeat the assessment and refine your observations until an image of your basic posture materializes. The ideal pos-

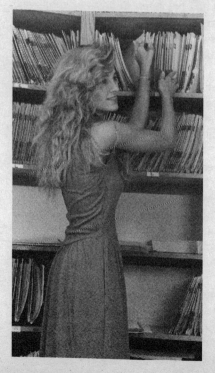

Monitor muscle tension during daily activity and take minibreaks to soothe muscles that are overused.

ture holds the body balanced and symmetrical. Where does yours need adjustment?

Ideally:
· The feet provide a comfortable base.
· The knees are slightly flexed.
· The buttocks are relaxed.
· The pelvis is square.
· The spine is supported by the pelvis.
· The shoulders are open and broad with your head resting comfortably over the shoulders.

By positioning the body into this posture, the muscles will be strengthened and balanced. In areas of imbalance, make postural adjustments and assess their effectiveness by the feedback you receive from your body. By closing your eyes and breathing abdominally, feedback is enhanced.

Postural correction while standing usually centers on:
· Are the feet comfortably apart and are you balanced firmly on the ground? If not, find the most stable position. Wearing shoes usually alters the center of gravity and balance.
· Are the knees hyperextended and locked into position? Practice flexing the knees slightly.
· Is the pelvis positioned under the spine and over the legs?
· Are the buttock muscles relaxed? Practice contracting the lower abdominal muscles to balance the pelvis and pull it under the lower spine. Abdominal breathing with your eyes closed is helpful to increase awareness of pelvic muscles.
· Is the spine elongated or stretched? Place the chin in a neutral position or slightly tucked back and practice lifting the spine. As you elongate, note how the curves in the lower and upper spine begin to straighten. Early on, the muscles may fatigue rather quickly. As you become aware

of fatigue, settle back into your routine posture. Repeat this exercise many times during the day to strengthen postural muscles and, ultimately, to maintain comfort in this posture for longer periods of time.

· Are there tender, stiff muscles in the upper chest, neck and shoulder areas? Because the majority of activities are done in front of the body, chest muscles tighten and shoulder muscles overstretch. Consequently, mechanical stresses roll the shoulders forward, sinking the posture over the chest.

Phase 4: Posture in Daily Activity

Regular exercise increases body awareness and strengthens the postural muscles to maintain balance. After several

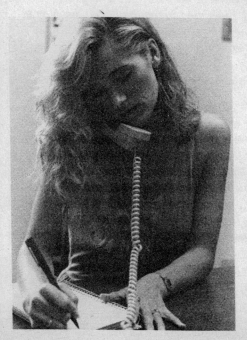

Holding the receiver of a phone between your head and shoulder while writing puts strain on the body.

weeks of doing exercises, put the newly developed posture into action. By analyzing your work environment, identify the physical strains associated with your job, such as holding the receiver of a phone between your head and shoulder while writing or typing or standing over a machine and doing repetitive activities for prolonged periods. As you go through your day, take frequent minibreaks to "listen" to the tension in your body and alter the activity that created it. Plan your work environment. Arrange your desk or work area to fit your needs and look for creative ways to renegotiate stressful tasks.

State of Alert

As a child, I watched families of gophers play in the field next to our house. We would sound a shrill whistle and watch the animals lift their heads and stiffen their bodies. They stood alert and vigilant until the threat had passed. Over the past few months, I noticed how I react the same way dozens of times each day. Whenever my boss calls my name, the kids argue or my spouse comes home from work, I assume a state of alert. And I hold that pattern much of the day. By keeping my muscles flexed much of the time, I have soreness in my neck and shoulders.

A prairie dog stands at attention to identify any threat.

Observe your behavior during work:
- How does your body cope with deadlines?
- How do you respond when your supervisor is around?
- How does your body deal with a difficult person?

The body reacts to different people and situations in various ways.

By learning about habits, posture and behavior may be modified. Place a posture picture or "relax" sign near the workstation as a reminder to assess posture and release the tension from the body frequently throughout the day.

Phase 5: Aerobic Exercise

Aerobic exercise is designed to increase the functional capacity of the heart and lungs. Excellent for reducing stress and improving heart function, aerobic exercise can worsen irritated, tender muscles if posture is inadequate. When muscles are tight and painful, stretching exercises may provide short-term relief. But if the muscles are overfatigued, they will often react with increased spasms.

Once the awareness and posture exercises have been mastered, the body is ready for aerobic exercise. An aerobic exercise program benefits almost everyone. The key is to find an exercise that is fun, sustainable and matches your level of physical conditioning.

Proper aerobic exercise strengthens both the static and phasic muscle systems, improves oxygen exchange in the lungs and makes the heart stronger. With exercise, muscles become more efficient at using oxygen. To be effective, aerobic exercise needs to be done on a daily or near-daily basis. Many top-notch aerobic exercise programs are available at YMCAs, YWCAs, health clubs or city park systems. Swimming is especially attractive because the sport utilizes a wide range of muscles and minimizes stress on any particular muscle group.

**AEROBIC POINTS ASSOCIATED WITH
COMMON PHYSICAL ACTIVITIES**

Walking	4 miles in 60 minutes = 11 points
	5 miles in 75 minutes = 14 points
Jogging	3 miles in 36 minutes = 11 points
	4 miles in 48 minutes = 15 points
	3 miles in 30 minutes = 14 points
Swimming	800 yards in 25 minutes = 6 points
	1,000 yards in 25 minutes = 10 points
	1,250 yards in 25 minutes = 14 points
Stationary Bike	at 35 mph = 1 point/3 minutes
Racquetball	10 points/60 minutes

Aerobic exercise is measured by aerobic points. A complete list of the aerobic points assigned to a given activity may be found in Kenneth Cooper's book, *The Aerobic Way.* The table above highlights popular forms of aerobic exercises. For maximum benefit, 60–65 aerobic points per week are recommended.

Choose exercises that increase body awareness and enable monitoring of physical fatigue. Often conditioning programs that emphasize pushing the body to the limit lead to injury. The health benefits of aerobic exercise are most noticeable for those progressing from a sedentary lifestyle to one that includes a modest degree of activity. Once conditioning is established, strenuous exercise goals are possible.

Getting Physically Fit

Walking is a simple way to condition the body and to prepare for more strenuous exercise. Physical fitness is a process. Begin with walking briskly, but comfortably for 15 minutes every day. Pace yourself or slow down if the body tires after 5 or 10 minutes. Then, add 2 to 5 minutes of walking each week until you can walk for a full 60 minutes. Measure the distance you cover in that time period. Ultimately, the goal is to walk 4 miles in 60 minutes. When this becomes easy, your body is ready to engage in any other form of aerobic exercise.

Sleep

Adequate sleep is a restorative activity that can prevent headaches. Recurrent headaches, however, often interfere with a stable sleep pattern. Headache sufferers may awaken in the morning feeling tired and sore.

To improve sleep, eliminate caffeine and establish a predictable sleep pattern. Sleep, like any other habit, requires consistency, including an established time to go to bed and a certain hour to wake up. The required number of hours of quality sleep varies between individuals. Generally, 6 to 9 hours of sleep is adequate.

Avoid large meals before bedtime. In the hour before sleep, engage in activities that relax the body, such as biofeedback, pleasurable reading or a warm bath. Evaluate your bed for comfort and a sense of security. Find a relaxed position where muscles are not strained. The pillow should not be too thick. Find a pattern for falling to sleep. Several deep relaxing breaths and a pleasant visualization induce slumber. If you awaken during the night, use the same formula to fall back to sleep. Almost everyone will have occasional restless nights, and if that happens, program yourself to look forward to the next night of good sleep.

Medications can assist sleep. Sleeping pills, however, can be addictive, cause headache transformation and block deeper stages of sleep that assure adequate restoration. When head pain interferes with sleep, tricyclic antidepressants in small doses often aid sleeping.

Tips for the Workplace

1) Organize your desk for comfort and ease.
2) Make sure your chair fits you: that your feet are on the floor, your back is supported and the height is adjusted to allow your arms to work comfortably.
3) Do not hold the phone receiver cocked in your neck. If you need to write or use your hands while on the phone, ask your employer for a headset.
4) Decorate your area to your taste. Make the workplace aesthetically pleasing. Bring pictures of your family or favorite activities.
5) Get up and move around frequently.
6) Avoid hanging around the coffeepot. Bring herbal teas or drink water with a slice of lime as a substitute for coffee.
7) Remember to breathe abdominally. Place a reminder to take two deep relaxing breaths in a prominent place in your workspace.
8) Have fun and develop a sense of humor about things that are stressful or not going exactly as you had planned.
9) Practice sharing responsibilities with your co-workers. Learn to manage time and avoid taking on more than you can do. This makes you successful at what you do and makes work more rewarding.
10) Learn to ask for help before you become overwhelmed.

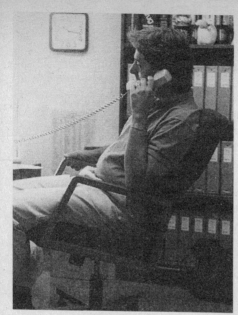

Your chair needs to fit you: your feet should rest on the floor and your back requires support.

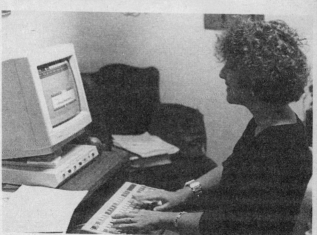

Your workstation needs to be the correct height to allow you to work easily and comfortably.

Sex

Sex and headaches are often thought of as the "not tonight, dear, I have a headache" syndrome. Gratifying sexual activity, however, reduces stress, enhances positive feelings and inspires a general sense of well-being. Many migraineurs report that engaging in sexual activity early in the course of a headache often aborts the attack. Making time for intimacy restores and nurtures the system.

Conclusion

Restorative activities optimize health. The body becomes more resilient and stronger. The world seems brighter and friendlier. Exercise improves body awareness and encourages an appreciation of the marvelous feedback system that maintains balance between the internal and external environments.

8

BIOFEEDBACK FOR HEADACHE CONTROL

What Is Biofeedback?

The nervous system constantly adjusts to demands of the environment and directs thousands of internal responses that maintain equilibrium. During change, the nervous system communicates new instructions to the body for restoring equilibrium. Information about how well the body adjusts to this change is fed back to the nervous system and refinements are made. This communication process is called *biofeedback,* life teaching itself to adjust to its environment.

Biofeedback is the way we learn most of our responses to the world. From riding a bicycle to shooting a basketball, the process of learning relies on the feedback between what we desire and how close we come to obtaining it. When the nervous system receives clear information about its responses, the process of learning is accelerated.

Science has capitalized on this by using devices that provide reliable information to the

BIOFEEDBACK LINKS THE BODY TO THE ENVIRONMENT.

nervous system about a desired response. For example, if a desired response is weight loss, a scale informs the body as to whether a new diet and exercise program are achieving fewer pounds.

Why Is Biofeedback
Important for Headache Control?

Migraineurs often have cold hands and feet. About 20 years ago, researchers noted that migraineurs generally had finger temperatures in the 70°F range, while those without headaches had finger temperatures in the 85°F range. Because migraine is believed to be a disorder of blood vessel control, researchers reasoned that headache sufferers might benefit from learning to increase their finger temperature. In a study, migraineurs were instructed to raise their finger temperature. A thermometer placed on the finger was used to monitor progress. The results were gratifying. Through the process of redirecting blood flow to the hands, finger temperature rose and the frequency of migraine attacks decreased. Since then, countless studies have demonstrated that thermal biofeedback (finger-warming) is one of the most effective means for preventing migraines.

How Useful Is
Biofeedback in Migraines?

Research utilizing thermal biofeedback in migraines has consistently demonstrated that 60 to 75 percent of headache sufferers reduce migraine attacks by at least 50 percent through practicing temperature biofeedback twice a day. Biofeedback is a powerful, safe mechanism for restoring a healthy balance to the nervous system. Over the years, biofeedback techniques have become more sophisticated, increasing the efficiency of the entire process.

How Do I Learn Biofeedback?

Biofeedback training is usually provided by a psychologist. Your physician or the local mental health association can recommend a psychologist with expertise in teaching biofeedback for headache relief. Generally, biofeedback training takes 5 or 6 sessions to learn the basics. In addition, daily practice is necessary to maximize its effectiveness. Psychologists who specialize in the treatment of headaches also teach coping strategies for managing life's tensions, especially learning to deal with the fear of future headaches and avoiding abusive patterns of medication usage. The psy-

Headache Spiral

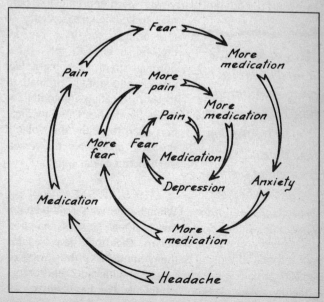

chologist works closely with the physician to provide more comprehensive management of headaches.

Learning Biofeedback

PAIN AND STRESS

Pain is one of the most stressful sensations for the nervous system to handle. Often signaling an emergency, pain activates the body to do whatever is necessary to stop the discomfort and avoid future painful encounters. As children, we probably learned what *hot* meant by getting burned. The memory of that painful experience protects us from touching things that are hot. In this way, pain protects the body from injury and helps the individual adjust more confidently to the surroundings. But if pain is not associated with a specific incident, the environment itself may become a source of uncertainty. Worry over when unpredictable pain may strike becomes a source of fear and, in the long run, increases stress. With this added burden, stress chemicals like adrenaline routinely circulate in the body, creating a potential for future headaches. Often medication, used to rectify this volatile situation, may serve to worsen the headache–fear spiral.

"My last headache started when I got a ticket for not stopping completely at a stop sign. Anything new, unusual or unplanned seems to cause a headache. I wish I would learn how to handle the unexpected better."

THE STRESS REACTION

When the nervous system identifies a threat, a stress reaction occurs. The body gears up for the emergency by increasing adrenaline and other stress chemicals. The heartbeat accelerates, breathing becomes shallow and rapid, the pupils dilate and blood is directed to the large muscles of the arms and legs. This is called the *fight-or-flight* response. The stress response is essential for battle or escape from a threatening situation. But if battle or escape is impossible, the stress response produces an imbalance in the internal chemical environment of the body. As the demands on the nervous system accumulate, the likelihood of a headache increases.

THE RELAXATION RESPONSE

The nervous system balances the stress response with other chemical messengers that communicate resolution of the threat. The body can relax. A sense of calm prevails and blood flow returns to the fingers, toes and digestive system. This relaxation response creates an internal environment resistant to headaches.

The relaxation response is assisted by learning techniques that maintain calm and security. Simply by interpreting events as predictable and understandable dampens the stress response. To reinterpret stress as challenge, transforms fear into determination. The eventual goal of the relaxation

See yourself on a beach, relaxed, one with nature.

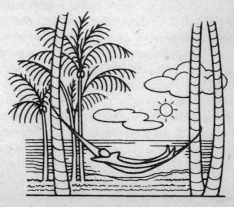

response is to remain calm even in the face of stressful conditions.

RETRAINING THE BODY'S RESPONSE

Retraining the nervous system to respond with relaxation instead of stress takes practice. Psychologists teach a variety of techniques to achieve this goal. By understanding the headache process and improving stress management, the headache threshold is protected. Relaxation techniques can change a picture of fear into one of control, ultimately preventing headaches. Biofeedback techniques are easy to learn and reinforce body responses that restore balance to the nervous system.

Thermal Biofeedback

The process of thermal biofeedback training begins with finding a quiet spot at home, free from interruptions. A finger thermometer provides the necessary feedback. Find a comfortable position and place the thermometer on the index finger. The bulb of the thermometer should rest on the fleshiest part of the fingertip. Secure the thermometer with tape. Record the finger temperature. Listening to soothing music or a relaxation audiotape assists finger-warming.

Place yourself in a comfortable position, either sitting or lying down. Uncross your arms and legs. Tell yourself you will not fall asleep, but will increase the finger temperature by 2 or 3 degrees after completing the exercise. While listening to the music or relaxation tape, close your eyes and begin to breathe slowly, using abdominal breathing techniques (see Chapter 7). Breathe in through your nose to a count of 4, hold the breath for 4 seconds and then exhale slowly through your mouth to a count of 8. Continue this pattern of breathing until the breath moves freely in and out of the lungs.

As you breathe in, say to yourself, "My hand . . ."; as you

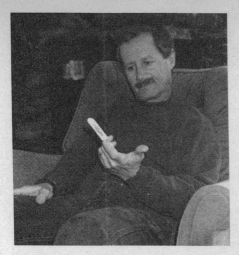

Thermal Biofeedback

exhale, say, ". . . is warm." "My hand is heavy and warm." Inventory each part of your body, until your entire body feels heavy and warm: "My fingers are heavy and warm"; "My legs are heavy and warm"; "My feet are heavy and warm." Then, "My breathing is calm and regular. My forehead is cool. My lungs breathe themselves."

Create a pleasant image in your mind. See yourself in a favorite spot in nature, such as on a lake or beach. Imagine the sun beaming heat into your fingers. At the same time, allow yourself to feel the calm, regular pulsations of your heartbeat carried to your fingers.

Clear your mind of interfering thoughts, worries and concerns by imagining a relaxing scene, such as a meadow, river or cloud formation, or by simply listening to the tape or music. Permit your thoughts to get lost in the images or music. Continue this exercise for about 20–30 minutes.

At the end of the exercise, record your finger temperature. If you have increased your finger temperature from 78°F to 81°F, for example, you will likely have a finger temperature of 81°F when you practice thermal biofeedback again. Practice twice a day: once in the morning and again in the evening. If the day has been particularly stressful, more practice sessions may be necessary.

With practice, a pattern of gradually increasing finger temperatures occurs and the finger temperature is higher at

---

The Message of Fireworks

I am a 39-year-old Japanese–American, married with two children, ages 5 and 2. My migraines used to occur several times a month. They would begin with a black spot appearing in the middle of what I was looking at. Flashing colored lights filled the space around the blackness. I was always afraid that I was going blind, even though I had had this for 10 years. The fear of blindness grew into panic and I felt like I had to run. I've bolted out of supermarkets and department stores because of these attacks. I felt like something was inside me that I couldn't get away from. Back then, I had no control over this and there was nothing to do but suffer until it went away.

My doctor suggested that I work with a psychologist.

During our sessions, I realized that I had difficulty expressing anger. During my childhood, my anger would hurt my parents. I felt guilty about having such bad feelings and I worried that they would not like me if I showed anger. Now, even as a married adult woman, I still was not expressing anger.

Another important discovery was that my aura

represented death to me. My father died about the same time my migraines began. There has been a lot of death in my family. My mother died 1 year ago and both my brothers are dead: one in an accident when I was 13 and the other from a heart condition 16 years ago. I feared that during one of these weird auras, I'd die, like the rest of my family.

Another stressor is my marriage. Frank is preoccupied with tennis and seems to care about nothing else, not even our children. I quit my job 6 years ago to be a full-time mother and now feel isolated from adult friends and betrayed by Frank. My isolation is compounded because I'm Oriental. I feel like a fraud to my culture because I don't know the Japanese language, customs or culture. My parents did not pass on our heritage. They wanted me to be "all-American."

With counseling and biofeedback training, I learned to relax and control these stresses. I identified people and events that upset me and I prepared myself to deal with them in a detached way. Eventually, I recognized that the fireworks of my aura were a message that meant I was not taking adequate care of myself. I was not exercising, eating properly, sleeping enough hours or dealing with my feelings. The aura has challenged me to see beyond my black-and-white logical approach to life and recognize its symbolic potential. I have begun to "see" and "work through" the blind spot of my aura rather than reject the visual disturbance as scary and strange.

the start of each practice session. This is a sign that the physiology of the body is being altered toward relaxation. If unwanted thoughts, worries or problems intrude during training, the finger temperature will not rise or may actually fall. If this occurs frequently, explore the thoughts or feelings that seem to block the relaxation response. At times, this is best done with a psychologist.

GOAL

Once the finger temperature rises to 96°F, the training period is over. The individual now has the power to direct blood into the fingers simply by willing or visualizing the fingers warming. No one has a natural finger temperature as high as 96°F. Achieving this level of warmth is a sign that physiological relaxation has been reached by voluntarily directing the blood flow into the fingers.

BIOFEEDBACK FOR PAIN CONTROL

If there is discomfort in other areas of the body, such as the muscles of the neck and shoulders, the biofeedback training can be modified to decrease the pain and tension. By

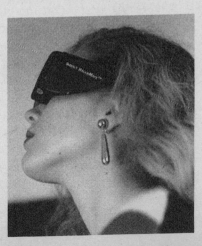

These glasses feature small strobe lights pulsating within the alpha frequency range to help promote relaxation.

concentrating on warming the area of discomfort, blood flow to the area is increased, providing more oxygen and glucose to the tissue. Waste products of excessive muscle tension, like lactic acid, are transported out and the muscles relax. This inevitably reduces pain and promotes a healing response. Because headaches may intensify by increasing blood flow to the head, this biofeedback exercise is reserved for areas of pain other than the head.

Other Types of Biofeedback

Biofeedback is a broad term that describes many techniques to change the awareness of the nervous system. Treatment-wise, there are basically three types of biofeedback: thermal, muscular and brain wave. Historically and statistically, thermal biofeedback is the most effective type in migraines. In special instances, however, other forms of biofeedback have been found effective in headache management.

EMG (Electromyographic) Biofeedback

At times, muscle tension and pain can be significant precipitators of the headache process. Individuals may react to stress by tightening muscles in the face, jaw, neck or shoulders. In these cases, modifying biofeedback to relax the muscles can relieve headaches.

The technique employed is called EMG biofeedback. Sensors that detect muscle tension are placed on the skin over specific muscles and provide feedback about the degree of tension in that muscle. This information is usually fed back as a digital readout or a tone, which is loud and high-pitched when the muscle is tense and becomes softer as the muscle relaxes.

During the initial training, a person learns to reduce muscle tension while resting. After this has been mastered, spe-

EMG Biofeedback

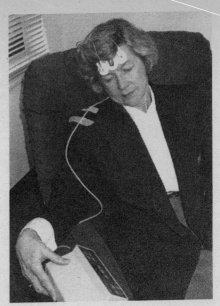

The brain map
(a 19-lead EEG)
measures the brain
wave activity to
determine whether
EEG biofeedback is
appropriate.
EEG biofeedback
requires the brain to
produce theta,
alpha or beta
waves in the part of
the brain where the
electrodes are
attached to the
scalp.

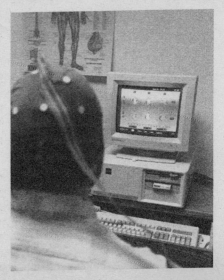

cific events which usually produce tension are reviewed with the goal of keeping the muscle relaxed. The sensors can be moved to other painful muscle groups as progress is made. Ultimately, these skills are transferred to daily life.

EMG biofeedback is useful in about 20 percent of headache cases. It is easy to learn, but requires more sophisticated equipment than does temperature biofeedback.

EEG (Electroencephalographic) Biofeedback

As the brain enters a more relaxed state, its electrical activity slows and calm prevails. Researchers have defined four states of electrical activity in the brain: beta, alpha, theta and delta. The most active state is beta, used for focused problem-solving. Alpha encompasses relaxation, when the body slows down, the muscles loosen and a sense of well-being pervades. During alpha activity or when the eyes are closed, the brain is absorbing a situation rather than reacting to it. Theta, a slower brain wave pattern associated with creative insight, occurs just before sleep and upon awakening, during the time of not being asleep yet not fully awake. Delta, the slowest brain activity, is characteristic of sleep.

EEG biofeedback uses sensors on the head to register electrical activity in the brain. Desired activity, usually alpha, is fed back to the person in the form of a tone or a picture on a monitor. With practice, a person may produce the desired activity voluntarily. By generating more alpha activity, the brain spends less time in an emergency mode.

EEG biofeedback helps change "thinking gears" for those who have difficulty quieting their thought processes. Those who "intellectualize" or are "worry warts," are often tense and manifest a predominance of beta. EEG biofeedback allows these individuals to switch into alpha and relaxation. It requires sophisticated machinery and is more expensive than other forms of biofeedback, but is very useful for about 10 percent of headache sufferers.

Conclusion

Biofeedback helps a person become more aware of reactions in the body. Through the process, insight is gained concerning how we react to situations and how to alter our responses in order to become more relaxed and healthy. Biofeedback is a safe, nondrug and effective way to prevent migraines, and imparts confidence and a sense of inner control. For many, it offers the choice between responding or reacting to the environment.

Relaxation/Visualization Exercise

Take a deep breath and slowly let it out. Take another deep breath and slowly let go. Two deep, cleansing breaths are a sign to our body that it is time to relax; it is time to let go. It is time to turn off the body and mind, just briefly, to go on a journey inward for knowledge and understanding.

Get in tune with your breathing as you breathe in peace, comfort and relaxation and you breathe out all negativity. Collect discomfort and breathe it out. Collect anger and breathe it out. Collect fear and breathe it out. Collect isolation and breathe it out. Collect all negative feelings and breathe them out.

With each breath, you can feel, sense and see yourself go deeper and deeper into relaxation as you become lighter and lighter. One breath at a time, one breath after another, with each breath you become twice as relaxed as you were the breath before.

Picture yourself standing underneath a waterfall of golden healing energy. The energy cascades over your head, swirls around your face and neck, goes down your chest and back and covers your body from head to toe. The energy sinks into your body through the pores of your skin and fills your body, from head to toe, with lightness, brightness and warmth.

As you fill your body with light, notice any areas of your body that may be heavy, dark, empty or pressured. Concentrate on filling these areas with light and dispelling the negativity from the body.

By filling your body with golden healing energy, the body becomes light, bright and warm enough to float. Picture yourself floating up, up into the sky, on a cloud toward the sun.

By filling the body with light and by covering the body with golden healing energy, the system is protected from negativity. Demands from people, events or situations can bounce off the layer of light that encircles the body. Inside, you are safe and secure from the drain of negativity. Even though turmoil may surround you, inside the buffer of light, you are calm, tranquil and serene.

Imagine a scene that is relaxing, your own private place: an island, beach, meadow, on a boat, in a hot-air balloon, riding on an eagle's wings, floating on an inner tube or fishing on the bank of a stream. Use this vista as a cue to put the entire body into a state of relaxation. Picture the scene in your mind immediately before giving a talk to a group or asking your boss for a raise in order to compose your nervous system and help you tap into your inner resources.

Record the relaxation exercise on an audiotape in your own voice. Listen to the tape, calm the body and warm the fingers to 96°F for 20 minutes twice a day, in the morning and the evening. In this way, the body, mind and spirit become balanced, freeing the nervous system from an accumulation of stress.

9

COPING SKILLS

Cognitive Restructuring

As toddlers, we incorporate guidelines from our parents, such as "brush your teeth before you go to bed" and "wash your hands before you eat." These become "should," "ought" or "must" as we grow up. Guilt may haunt us whenever we fail to live up to these rules. At times, children receive the message that they displease their parents because they do not live up to these expectations. These perceptions, truthful or misguided, may go through the mind without the person realizing that negativity is setting up the individual for defeat, sadness and disappointment.

To discover whether negative self-talk unknowingly affects you, listen to what you tell yourself when you make a mistake. Is it "I'll do better next time" or "I never do anything right"? If you are plagued by negativity, you can learn to replace the disparaging remarks with positive messages. Among headache sufferers, five frequent pessimistic self-evaluations are:

NEGATIVE SELF-TALK	AFFIRMATIONS
1. I am bad, fat, ugly, stupid, no good.	1. I am good.
2. There is something wrong with me.	2. I am me.
3. I can never please my spouse, children, parents, boss.	3. I forgive myself for being imperfect.
4. My life is a mess.	4. Headaches are manageable.
5. I should take care of everyone and everything.	5. I deserve health and harmony.

Case Studies

1. VALUE OF SELF

"I am an executive secretary. I have to look my best. I get my hair done every week and spend a couple of hours each morning with makeup and hairdo. I take pride in my wardrobe and I want to look professional whenever I leave the house. But these headaches that I have almost every day are making it nearly impossible for me to be pleasant and look good. I have no patience; I cannot tolerate incompetency. I'm as hard on the office staff as my boss is on me. But the operation runs smoothly. I eat lunch at my desk, if I get a chance. I get a lot of work done, but I don't have much of a life outside the office. My husband and I are exhausted by the end of the week; we just lie around all weekend. And then it's back to the grind again."

Negative Self-talk: I am not good enough.
Affirmation: I am good.

Identifying the negative phrase that a person says to him- or herself is the first step toward transforming the message to a positive one. Each time the person catches him- or herself saying an antagonistic statement, he or she needs to replace it with an affirmation. Eventually, with practice, the individual will be governed by an optimistic attitude.

2. SELF-JUDGMENT

"My father had headaches. He would cloister himself in the bedroom and cry out in pain. He suffered tremendously for as long as I can remember and then he died of a headache. I worry that my headaches will become that bad, that something is very wrong with me. I doubt if anything can help this pain in my head. It won't go away. It's like a big black cloud hanging over my head. When will it become too much for me to handle? When will I give up and stop fighting?"

Negative Self-talk: There is something wrong with me.
Affirmation: I am me.

Once the headache becomes controlled, life is no longer as gloomy. This man's father did not ask for help and as a result, suffered alone. But, he did not predestine his family to the misery he suffered. We all have choices. Suffering in silence rarely brings relief. Every individual lives his or her own life, including our own family members.

3. I AM WHAT I DO

"I'm lucky because I've been able to stay home to care for my kids. I keep a spotless house and fix a hot meal every night; sometimes at noon I deliver a hot lunch to my kids at school. I bake bread from scratch and in the wintertime, there's always a pot of soup simmering on the stove. My question is, why can't I make my family happy? The clothes the kids want for school are always the ones in the hamper. I don't press my husband's shirts to his liking. They want more variety in the suppers I serve. My mother says I don't call her enough, even though I talk to her at least once a day. I apologize for not having the right change at the store.

"Now my headaches won't leave me alone. The pain is killing me. There's a part of me that always had to please everyone. Now I can't do anything for anyone, not even myself. I can't please anyone, not even my own body."

Negative Self-talk: I can never please my spouse, children, parents, boss.
Affirmation: I forgive myself for being imperfect.

To please others, we need to please ourselves first. By allowing others to treat us like a doormat, we invite mistreatment. We try harder to meet others' expectations, only to be confronted with their disappointment in us. The first step in freeing ourselves from this spiral of abuse is to admit we are not perfect. Each person is responsible for his or her happiness. Dissatisfaction points out the need for change. Complaining individuals need to listen to their problems with others as indicators of what they need to alter in themselves.

4. LIFE IS OUT OF CONTROL

"I used to spend 3 or 4 days in bed, blinds drawn and lights out. I was hiding from life. I'd look in the mirror and I'd see an ugly, repulsive person. Pain does that. I wonder if I can ever feel beautiful again."

Negative Self-talk: My life is a mess.
Affirmation: Headaches are manageable.

"Now I know there's a recipe to my headaches:
- a little lack of sleep, usually less than 6 hours;
- a dash of monosodium glutamate (MSG); and
- more than two glasses of red wine (tyramine).

"These ingredients set me up to get a headache:
- if my period starts; or
- if I argue with my husband.

"I usually can control the onset of a headache with relaxation if I:
- get eight hours of sleep;
- avoid MSG; and
- avoid red wine.

"If a headache strikes, I know I can get rid of it within an hour by using my medication and doing my biofeedback exercises."

5. JUSTIFICATION FOR EXISTENCE

"My headaches started when I was 12. I was babysitting for a neighbor. The little girl was asleep in her room when a delivery man came to the door with a package. Because I had to sign for the item, I went to find a pen. When I returned to the livingroom, he was inside with the front door shut behind him. He said he wouldn't hurt me if I sat in the chair and was quiet. He fondled my whole body. I didn't move; I didn't shout at him. I never told anybody. I felt dirty and ashamed. Why did I let him have his way? I'm still angry with myself. Since then, my headaches paralyze me. I keep trying to prove to everyone that I am good. I take care of my parents; they've moved in with us. I help my husband with his painting business by doing the bookkeeping. I teach my kids at home. I volunteer at church. I visit nursing homes and bring the residents little gifts that I've made. But my headaches are getting worse."

Negative Self-talk: I should take care of everyone and everything.
Affirmation: I deserve health and harmony.

Headache relief begins with caring for yourself. Caretakers give to others until there is nothing left inside. Then, they can give to no one, especially themselves. Each of us needs to nurture our own health and pursue happiness. We then become models for others on how to achieve what everyone wants. The first step is believing that we deserve health and harmony. After an individual has suffered trauma, professional help may be necessary to release the negative attitudes and to plan a strategy for a more productive way of life.

Assertiveness Training

Whenever a person feels guilty, anxious or ignorant in the company of a certain individual, he or she is probably being manipulated by that person. The first question to ask oneself is, "do I deserve to feel guilty, anxious or ignorant?"

HEADACHE

Ever Present
In the wings
On the stage
At centerstage

Seldom
An opening
An intermission
A finale

Sometimes
Vibrato
Crescendo
Cacophony

Usually
Immeasurable
Endless
Boundless

Always
Perplexing
Distressing
Debilitating

Forever
Tolerated
Managed
Endured

EVER-PRESENT HEADACHE
by Maty Wright, 1993

The Power of "No"

If not, then you are being asked to do something you don't want to do. The second question is, "do you want to do what is being asked of you?"

If not, then say "no." To many individuals, "no" means rejection, abandonment or an invitation to the other person to become angry. Practice saying "no" in unimportant situations as preparation for saying "no" under significant circumstances.

"I am a unit secretary on a hospital ward and my headaches became so bad that I could not work. Medicine made me sleepy and draggy and interfered with my work. I was at my wit's end. My doctor referred me to a psychologist for biofeedback. She taped a portable thermometer to my finger and began asking me questions about my life. She noticed that my finger temperature continued to rise when I talked about my husband, kids, parents, even my stress at work. But when she asked me about my sister, my finger temperature nosedived into the 70s. I didn't realize that two of the nurses who were causing me problems reminded me of my sister, who has always competed with me. Those nurses, like my sister, are very demanding and treat me like a slave instead of a person. I was afraid I'd blow up at them at work, like I usually do to my sister whenever I see her. I didn't want to lose control; that would mean they would win, get the best of me. We practiced saying "no" to both nurses. It probably sounds silly, but I have trouble saying "no" to anyone, much less someone

who makes me feel inferior. I would play the nurse and the psychologist would say "no," and then she would act like the nurse (and my sister) and I could finally say "no" without crying.

"At work, I couldn't believe my ears when I told the nurse, "no, I cannot work through lunch"; "no, I cannot do what you want until I finish what I am currently working on"; "no, I cannot run down to the cafeteria and get you a snack." I overheard one of the nurses say that I've changed a lot since I took sick leave and the other commented that my headaches must really be bad since I'm acting so independent. But the reverse was true; I didn't have a single headache when I was standing up for myself.

"The ultimate challenge was over the Thanksgiving holiday, when I was with my sister. I said "no" to her and to my surprise, she was not angry or hurt. We got along fine, probably the best ever. Finally we see each other as sisters rather than competitors."

IDENTIFYING GOALS

After finding out what you do not want to do, the next feat is discovering what you want. Once a goal is identified, you have a definite path to follow.

"I've always wanted to be a potter. I love the feel of clay. My husband thought the idea was ridiculous. What will I do with the pots when they're finished? Will they be worth anything? Who will want to buy them? He wanted me to help him on the farm. He milks 86-head of cattle twice a day. His folks live next door; his mother milks in the morning and his dad does the chores in the evening. He wanted to know why I couldn't be satisfied being the wife of a dairy farmer.

"I felt foolish and selfish. What made me think I'd be any good at making pottery? But at the feed store, I saw an ad for a noncredit pottery course to be taught at night at the high school. When I told David, he agreed to let me go, but I'd have to find a babysitter.

"The class was small—only four of us—but the instructor encouraged us to be creative and invent our own designs. He said I had talent. To make a long story short, I got a wheel and worked on pottery at night after the chores were done. As the wheel spun around, my headaches left. I took my pots to a gallery in the city and they began to sell them, much to everyone's surprise. Since I'm making money and still doing the chores, David is happy. I haven't told him yet that I'm planning a show in a metropolitan area 4 hours away. But he sees that I am floating on a cloud and I am a joy to have around, so he's not complaining even if he doesn't understand what I find in pottery."

Journaling

Headache sufferers often assume that they feel only one emotion—pain. The finer differentiations of feeling are numbed under the misery of a migraine. But as an individual reclaims his or her life by controlling headaches, emotions surface. To reacquaint oneself to sensations, a Feeling and Dream Journal is a way to plot the progress toward greater sensitivity and understanding of the daily fluctuations in mood. Without a record of these nuances, the subtle transformation of perception, response, motivation and energy level will be lost in the adventure of a new lease on life.

FEELING JOURNAL

Date	Occurrence	Feeling	Response	Result
EXAMPLE:				
1/1/94	*Phone call from Sandy*	*Happiness/ gratitude*	*Wrote letter to her*	*Friendship rekindled*
2/14/94	*No gift*	*Disappointment*	*Told him of anger, hurt*	*Surprised me with tickets to play*

DREAM JOURNAL

Title of dream	Feeling	Message	Application in life
EXAMPLE:			
Friendly sharks	*Fear/humor*	*Cannot count on appearances*	*See things through; don't assume without checking things out*

BEARING PAIN

When pain gets more than I can bear,
Then I look up and say a prayer.
When I reach out in my despair,
Then I "Thank God" for being there.

When it seems there is "no way,"
He calms my fears and dries my tears,
Then helps me through another day.

by Shirley Smith, April 1992

10

THE TREATMENT OF HEADACHES

Medications

Unpredictable headaches stalk their victims, producing pain, disability and fear. Even after diet and lifestyle are modified, headaches can occur. During these attacks, medication is often necessary. Successfully utilized, medication often brings prompt relief of symptoms and imparts a sense of control over the headache process. This success allows the fear of future attacks to diminish and renews confidence that life is more manageable.

Headaches as a Signal

A headache attack is a warning, a signal that the body is not balanced. The internal chemistry is out-of-line. The goal of treatment is to assist the nervous system to regain and maintain its normal balance. Symptoms associated with a headache are like a set of instructions, directing changes necessary for relief. During a migraine, for instance, an individual seeks rest and withdraws from further stimulation of the nervous system. Sensitivity to light, sound, touch and smell causes the person to recoil from additional input to the nervous system until the body again achieves equilibrium. Paying attention to these signals assists the nervous system with regaining equilibrium.

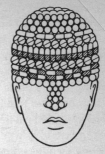

Face of Pills

When a headache attack occurs, the natural tendency is to fight the pain, keep going and not give in to the distress. Panic may set in when the pain and suffering become too much. But by learning when and how to take medication, the devastation of headaches is reduced. By recognizing the wisdom of the body, migraine treatment becomes more successful.

Medications Assist Rebalancing

Medications are divided into two general categories: 1) those used to thwart or stop acute attacks; and 2) preventatives or prophylactics that reduce the frequency and severity of attacks. Some acute medications diminish symptoms, while others accelerate the corrective process. Preventative medications protect the headache threshold.

Headache Control Plan

Devise a headache control plan before an attack occurs. Simple measures can augment the success of treatment. These include: 1) know your medication, especially how and when to use it; 2) rest for at least 30 minutes at the beginning of headache treatment; 3) withdraw from aggravating people, places or things; 4) put your

A HEADACHE CONTROL PLAN HELPS CONQUER FEAR AND PANIC.

health needs first and the demands of the situation second; and 5) plan a back-up strategy if the initial treatment does not work. Much like a fire drill, a headache procedure creates a sense of control which de-emphasizes fear and panic.

Response to medications varies from person to person or even headache to headache. Finding an effective medication program requires a partnership with the physician. Successful medical treatment is often a process of educated trial-and-error. By working with the physician and monitoring treatment response, the process is refined and a beneficial program can almost always be found.

Medication for Acute Treatment

Many different medications are available for acute treatment of headaches. Some, like narcotics, are designed to numb pain; others relieve symptoms like nausea or muscle tension; and a few reverse the migraine process.

Medication for Acute Treatment of Migraines

SUMATRIPTAN

(Imitrex) and **ergotamines** reverse migraines by interacting with specific parts of nerve cells to restore normal equilibrium. They do this by mimicking an important natural brain chemical called serotonin, which decreases during the migraine process. These medications work like a lock and key, with the medication being a key that fits into a lock on the nerve or blood vessel wall. This interaction "unlocks" a response that restores equilibrium. By replacing serotonin at specific places in the nervous system, these medications promote a return to normal functioning.

Serotonin, given during a migraine, can bring relief. In-

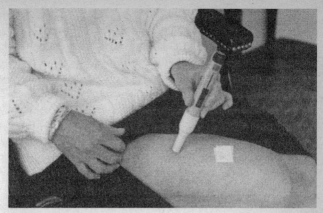

By using a self-injection device, sumatriptan (Imitrex) is delivered quickly and easily into the fat tissue of the thigh for relief of migraines.

jected into the bloodstream, however, it acts like a "master key" that activates many different serotonin receptors. As a result, many unwanted and even dangerous side effects can occur. Ergotamines also stimulate receptors beyond those necessary to relieve migraines. By contrast, sumatriptan is highly specific in its lock and key activity and stimulates the receptors more directly involved in the migraine process.

Sumatriptan (Imitrex/Canada: Imigran): Sumatriptan is a newly approved drug for the treatment of migraines. It is the most studied of all antimigraine drugs. By mimicking serotonin, sumatriptan activates specific receptors in blood vessels and nerve endings around the brain. These activated receptors rapidly stop the inflammation around blood vessels involved in the migraine process and shrink stretched blood vessels. The nerves carrying the pain message become less irritable and more resistant to the pain message.

Demonstrated in several large research studies worldwide, sumatriptan effectively relieves 70 to 90 percent of acute migraine attacks. In addition, the medication lessens nausea as well as light and sound sensitivity. Perhaps as important as ameliorating migraine symptoms, many migraineurs report a prompt return to normal functioning.

Sumatriptan acts rapidly. Within 30 minutes of an injection of the medication, 50 percent of migraineurs experience easement of pain. Within 90 minutes, 80 to 90 percent have relief of pain and other associated symptoms. Almost 70 percent of migraineurs with moderate to severe attacks return to daily activity.

Sumatriptan is available in the United States as a self-injection system and a pill. The self-injection device holds a syringe containing medication, and with the push of a button, the injection is delivered into the fat tissue between the skin and the muscle of the thigh. Easy to use, the self-injection system has been found to produce less injection-site pain than when given by doctors or nurses.

The oral tablet is almost as effective as the injection at relieving migraine symptoms but takes longer to work. Most find relief within two hours. The recommended starting dose is 25 milligrams which can be repeated in two hours if needed. Up to 300 milligrams can be taken within 24 hours but no single dose should exceed 100 milligrams. Oral sumatriptan is particularly effective for migraine attacks that develop slowly without nausea or vomiting. The tablet also effectively treats migraines that return following successful treatment with an injection of sumatriptan. This is important since migraine symptoms return in about 40 percent of attacks treated by injection.

SIDE EFFECTS

The side effects associated with sumatriptan consist of burning or redness where the medicine is injected, flushing, numbness, and tingling, especially in the head and neck area. These side effects generally occur within 10 minutes of an injection and last for less than 30 minutes. Oral administration may produce the same side effects but generally less often and with less intensity. There have been very few serious adverse reactions associated with sumatriptan usage.

Sumatriptan has some effect on the blood vessels outside the head. Rarely, disturbances in the blood vessels of the heart have been noted. In individuals with certain heart problems, sumatriptan should be avoided or used only under close physician supervision. It should be avoided in people with uncontrolled elevation of blood pressure, blood vessel diseases or a rare type of heart pain called Printzmetal's angina. People with liver disease or using medications, such as, ergotamine or MAO inhibitors should seek an alternative treatment. For most migraineurs, however, sumatriptan is a safe treatment.

Ergotamines

BELLERGAL-S (phenobarbital–ergotamine–belladonna)
CAFERGOT (ergotamine–caffeine)
ERGOSTAT/ERGOMAR (ergotamine)
WIGRAINE (ergotamine–caffeine)

A cornerstone in migraine treatment, ergotamines were first used in 1927. Early pioneering work by Harold Wolff and John Graham demonstrated that these drugs constricted blood vessels believed to be involved in the migraine process. Recent research has elaborated on this process, noting that in addition to contracting blood vessels, ergotamines stimulate serotonin receptors, offering more complete migraine relief.

AVAILABLE IN DIFFERENT FORMS, ERGOTAMINE DOSAGES CAN EASILY BE INDIVIDUALIZED.

Ergotamines are effective in migraines, especially when they are given early in the course of the attack. Because they may induce nausea, a medication for nausea, such as meto-clopramide (Reglan), may also be taken.

VARIOUS FORMULATIONS

Response to ergotamines is highly individual, and finding the right dose and best way to use these compounds are paramount. Ergotamines are available in different forms, allowing for individualization of administration.

If nausea or loss of appetite are present during a migraine, indicating that oral medications would not be absorbed well, ergotamine preparations that are dissolved under the tongue or used as a rectal suppository are available. Rectal suppositories are particularly useful because the dose can be easily individualized. There is a simple test to determine the proper amount of an ergotamine rectal suppository that is tolerated without side effects. It is best to do this test on a nonmigraine day. Begin with one-fourth of a rectal suppository, and if after 30 minutes there is no nausea, then add another one-fourth suppository and so on, until one experiences only slight nausea or is tolerating a whole suppository. When a migraine occurs, a treatment dosage slightly less than that noted to produce side effects will be a well-tolerated starting dosage.

SIDE EFFECTS

The common side effects of ergotamines are nausea, vomiting and muscle cramps. Because ergotamines constrict blood vessels, circulation problems may arise in individuals who are sensitive to these drugs, take them in excessive doses or for prolonged periods of time. If blood vessels in the arms or legs become too constricted, extremities may feel painfully cold, numb or tingly. The pulse in the wrist or foot may become weak. If ergotamine intake continues, the resulting lack of circulation can produce serious consequences.

Ergotamines are not used in people with heart disease, blood vessel disease, uncontrolled high blood pressure or Prinzmetal's angina. They are also avoided in those with significant liver or kidney disease or during pregnancy, as they can restrict blood to the growing baby. Ergotamines can cause dependency and lead to rebound headaches. Dependency is possible if ergotamines are used on a daily or near-daily basis. If a severe headache results after prolonged use of ergotamines, then rebound headaches from ergotamines are the likely cause. Except under direct supervision of a physician knowledgeable in the treatment of headaches, ergotamines should not be taken on a daily basis. Experience suggests that daily use of ergotamines over an extended period of time is likely to lead to complications. Instead, ergotamines are most effective when dosages are individualized and used early in the course of a migraine.

DHE–45 (DIHYDROERGOTAMINE)

DHE–45 is a somewhat unique ergotamine. As a migraine alleviator, DHE works by stimulating serotonin receptors. DHE offers strong interaction with serotonin receptors specific for headache relief and some experts feel it may not constrict blood vessels as much as other ergotamines. DHE is available as an injection and can be given as a shot into the muscle or directly in the bloodstream. Patients can be taught to give DHE injections into the muscle for home use.

DHE successfully soothes a migraine attack within 1 hour for up to 70 percent of migraine patients. Because nausea may be a side effect, medications that subdue an upset stomach can be given in combination with DHE. This increases DHE's effectiveness and minimizes the queasiness.

DHE is also effective in breaking through chronic daily headache patterns, including those that are the result of medication rebound. In these cases, hospitalization is sometimes required. DHE is given intravenously every 8 hours until the headache cycle is disrupted and then the medication is slowly withdrawn. Often DHE is continued as an intermittent self-injection to stop future attacks.

The risks and side effects associated with DHE are essentially the same as with other ergotamines. DHE is not indicated in persons with heart disease, uncontrolled high blood pressure, blood vessel disease, serious kidney or liver disease or during pregnancy or lactation. Use of DHE on a chronic basis should be monitored closely by a physician.

Drugs that Block Inflammation

ASPIRIN
ORUDIS (ketoprofen)
TOLECTIN (tolmetin)
MOTRIN/ADVIL (ibuprofen)
LODINE (etodolac)
TORADOL (ketorolac)
NAPROSYN (naproxen)
FELDENE (piroxicam)
MECLOMEN (meclofenamate)

During the migraine process, inflammation erupts around the blood vessel walls in the head, generating much of the pain. By inhibiting this inflammation, the pain message going to the brain is blocked. A number of drugs are effective in stopping this inflammatory reaction and provide a degree of relief from migraine pain. Commonly, these drugs are used to treat arthritis.

These drugs are usually well-tolerated and can be taken orally, making them convenient when nausea or stomach problems are not serious. When prescribed dosages are followed, few side effects arise. Out of desperation, however, a person may take extra amounts of the medication. In these cases,

MEDICATION TAKEN IN ANTICIPATION OF A HEADACHE WORSENS THE PROBLEM.

significant stomach difficulties, and at times, ulcers may develop. Kidney and liver injury is also possible.

Some of these agents may be available without a prescription and may be viewed as not being "real" medications. This misperception may lead to overuse and potentially serious side effects. Also, because of their availability, these medications may be taken in anticipation of a headache. This misuse can worsen the headache problem (see Chapter 3).

ASPIRIN

A simple and effective acute treatment for migraines is aspirin. Take 2 Alka-Seltzer tablets (Alka-Seltzer contains aspirin) in warm water with 1 aspirin tablet. Aspirin in this form is absorbed from the stomach more rapidly. Taking aspirin early in the headache process increases its effectiveness. Caffeine combined with aspirin boosts its potency and drinking coffee with aspirin is an inexpensive way to knock out a headache. Many over-the-counter remedies, such as Excedrin, contain caffeine to capitalize on this interaction. Keep in mind that the addition of caffeine on a frequent basis also increases the risk of headache rebound.

NONSTEROIDAL ANTI-INFLAMMATORY DRUGS (NSAIDS)

Nonsteroidal anti-inflammatory drugs or NSAIDs are commonly used to treat the inflammation of arthritis and can block the inflammatory process associated with migraines as well. The dose necessary in headaches is often higher than that used in arthritis. Most of these medications have about the same effectiveness, but individual responses to the different NSAIDs may vary. If one NSAID fails to provide relief, try another before deciding that this class of medication is not effective.

Toradol is a nonsteroidal that is available as a tablet and an injection. Injectable Toradol has more predictable absorption, especially when nausea is present, and has been demonstrated as a moderately successful treatment in migraines.

NSAID medications can also be used for prevention when migraine attacks are associated with predictable, recurrent events, such as menses, coitus or exercise. Administering these compounds prior to this time of vulnerability can deter or diminish headache attacks.

SIDE EFFECTS

These drugs are generally well-tolerated. They can cause irritation of the stomach lining and even ulcers. If stomach upset occurs, consult your physician. NSAIDs can also be toxic to the liver, bone marrow and kidney, especially when used over long periods of time. Some of these drugs can, on occasion, cause headaches.

> NSAIDS DO NOT AFFECT MENTAL ALERTNESS.

To date, there is no convincing evidence that NSAIDs lead to rebound or transformed headache patterns, although chronic daily administration of these compounds should probably be avoided. NSAIDs generally do not affect mental alertness, making the medication compatible with efficient daily functioning.

Drugs that Treat Symptoms

ANALGESIC COMBINATION PRODUCTS

FIORINAL (butalbital–aspirin-caffeine)
EXCEDRIN (aspirin–caffeine)
MIDRIN (isometheptene–dichloralphenazone–
    acetaminophen)
ESGIC-PLUS (butalbital–acetaminophen–caffeine)
DARVOCET/DARVON (propoxyphene)

Numerous medications combine analgesics (pain-killers), sedatives, caffeine and/or compounds that contract blood vessels and are useful for headache treatment. Excedrin (aspirin–caffeine), Fiorinal (butalbital–aspirin–caffeine) and Midrin (isometheptene–dichloralphenazone–acetaminophen) are popular examples. Even though there are few well-controlled studies that support the effectiveness of these combination products for headache relief, they have proven their worth over time for many headache sufferers. Caffeine and isometheptene (the chemical in Midrin) constrict blood vessels, which may be beneficial in terminating headache symptoms. In patients where anxiety is a significant component of the headache attack, sedatives, such as butalbital, may be useful.

SIDE EFFECTS

Combination products yield side effects common to each component of the product. They are generally well-tolerated, but sedation is common. As a word of caution, when pain medication is combined with caffeine and/or sedatives and used daily, even in modest quantities, the risk increases for dependency and chronic daily headache transformation (see Chapter 3).

NARCOTIC ANALGESICS

DEMEROL (meperidine)
LORCET (hydrocodone–acetaminophen)
TYLOX/CANADA: OXYCOCET (oxycodone–acetaminophen)
MORPHINE
PERCOCET/PERCODAN (oxycodone–acetaminophen–aspirin)
TYLENOL #3 OR #4 (codeine–acetaminophen)
SYNALGOS-DC (dihydrocodeine–aspirin–caffeine)
FIORINAL WITH CODEINE (butalbital–aspirin–caffeine–codeine)
VICODIN (hydrocodone–acetaminophen)

Traditionally, narcotic pain relievers have been a mainstay treatment for severely disabling headaches and are effective in some cases. Since narcotics can lead to addiction and have side effects that impair function, their routine use should not be encouraged. Narcotics are valuable for infrequent attacks of headache which are not easily controlled by other therapies or when there are reasons prohibiting the use of other therapies. Because narcotics can increase nausea and vomiting, they are frequently combined with drugs that prevent nausea. This combination increases the sedation of narcotics and can impair judgment, coordination and the ability to drive. Narcotics are also one of the most potent chemicals to cause rebound headaches.

Stadol and Nubain have recently been promoted for use in acute treatment of migraines. They are somewhat different chemically from narcotics, but by and large, have the same advantages and disadvantages.

Antinausea Drugs

Medications commonly used to suppress nausea also relieve migraines. Two classes commonly used are antidopaminergic drugs and antihistamines. Even though these medications by themselves can, at times, effectively stop headaches, they are more commonly used in combination with other migraine treatments. Combining these medications with other migraine drugs increases the effectiveness of each individual medication.

Through the relief of nausea, these drugs also help the intestinal tract absorb other migraine medications. Antinausea medications are available as a pill, suppository or injection.

ANTIDOPAMINERGIC DRUGS
REGLAN (metoclopramide)
COMPAZINE/CANADA: PRORAZINE/STEMETIL (prochlorperazine)
THORAZINE/CANADA: LARYAETIL (chlorpromazine)

Compazine (prochlorperazine) and Thorazine (chlorpromazine) have strong antimigraine effects. In a double-blind study, prochlorperazine (Compazine) relieved migraines in 60 percent of the cases. Used in combination with DHE, the effectiveness increased to 70 percent. Chlorpromazine has an even stronger antimigraine effect. Used in emergency departments under close supervision as an intravenous treatment, the medication relieved migraines in 90 percent of the cases. Reglan (metoclopramide) has less of an antimigraine effect, but in general, is better tolerated and highly effective in relief of migraine-associated nausea.

SIDE EFFECTS

Potential side effects of these medications are significant. Compazine and Thorazine may produce sedation, restlessness, intense anxiety, a drop in blood pressure and, sometimes, uncontrolled muscle movements. Tardive dyskinesia is a permanent uncontrollable movement disorder of muscles in the face, tongue and elsewhere. Though rare, this side effect may occur even with brief exposure to this class of drugs. Reglan is less likely to cause these side effects and is frequently used in conjunction with other treatment medications.

ANTIHISTAMINES

BENADRYL (diphenhydramine)
VISTARIL/CANADA: ATARAX/MULTIPAX (hydroxyzine)
PHENERGAN (promethazine)
PERIACTIN (cyproheptadine)

Numerous antihistamines may be helpful in treatment of acute migraines. Diphenhydramine (Benadryl), hydroxyzine (Vistaril) and promethazine (Phenergan) are commonly employed. They provide sedation, relieve nausea and enhance the effect of many pain medicines. Cyproheptadine (Periactin) is commonly used in children.

Typically, antihistamines are well-tolerated though often

PREVENTATIVE DRUGS MAY
DECREASE HEADACHE
FREQUENCY BY MORE
THAN 50 PERCENT.

sedating. Rarely, they cause disturbances of cardiac rhythm and potentiate seizures. The probability of side effects is increased by other medications, such as narcotics, alcohol and barbituates.

OTHER

TRAMADOL (Ultram) is a newly-developed pain reliever for moderate to moderately severe pain that may be useful in treating a variety of headache types. It presumably works by delaying the breakdown of certain brain chemicals important in pain relief. Tramadol is not likely to produce dependence but whether it can cause migraine transformation is unknown. Most common side effects include dizziness, nausea, malaise, and stomach-related problems. The exact role of tramadol in treatment of headache remains to be clarified.

Medication for Acute Treatment of Cluster Headaches

OXYGEN
DHE
ERGOTAMINES
SUMATRIPTAN

A cluster headache is an abrupt headache and does not last as long as a migraine. It is very severe, however, and demands rapid-acting medication. It is important that during a cluster period, alcohol, naps, disruption of sleep patterns and volatile chemicals be avoided, as they can all precipitate cluster attacks. Also, avoiding narcotics prevents cluster headaches from becoming more resistant to treatment.

The best therapy is inhaled oxygen. Breathing 100 percent oxygen through a face mask with a normal respiratory rate for up to 20 minutes will stop most cluster headaches. Since these headaches frequently awaken an individual from sleep, having an oxygen supply setup at the bedside can be of great value.

Ergotamines, including DHE, can also be employed to treat acute attacks of cluster. Ergotamines that are absorbed under the tongue ensure more rapid access to the bloodstream. DHE is also effective when given as an injection into the muscle or directly into the bloodstream.

Sumatriptan, given as an injection under the skin, has also been reported to be effective in relieving cluster headaches. It is used to treat acute attacks of cluster headaches in many countries outside the United States. Sumatriptan, however, is not approved by the FDA for use in cluster headache in the United States.

Medication for Acute Treatment of Tension-type Headaches

SIMPLE PAIN MEDICATIONS
ASPIRIN
TYLENOL (acetaminophen)

MUSCLE RELAXANTS
SOMA (carisoprodol)
PARAFON FORTE (chlorzoxazone)
FLEXERIL (cyclobenzaprine)

COMBINATION PRODUCTS
MIDRIN (cyclobenzaprine)
FIORINAL/FIORICET
ESGIC-PLUS

NSAIDS (*see page 131*)

Tension-type headaches do not typically cause the disability and suffering associated with migraines or clusters, and are generally treated by simpler means. Frequently, rest combined with simple pain medicines, such as aspirin, ibuprofen or other NSAIDs, is adequate. Occasionally, muscle relaxants or stronger combination products are employed, especially if the tension headache is more severe or chronic. Heat, ice rubs, spray and stretch techniques, exercise and Transcutaneous Electrical Stimulation (TENS) can be valuable supportive therapies.

Preventative Treatment of Headaches

PROPHYLACTIC PHARMACOLOGY

Prophylactic or preventative medication is taken regularly to prevent headache attacks. Prescribed for frequent disabling headaches or when acute therapies are inadequate, these medications rarely prevent all attacks. Generally, preventative drugs are considered successful when headaches decrease in frequency by at least 50 percent. They may be useful to gain control of a headache pattern during the challenge of altering lifestyle habits. Prophylaxis is often a trade-off between benefits and side effects. Many medications are effective in headache prevention, but response to various prophylactic medications varies widely. Finding the most effective medication and proper dosage is largely a process of trial-and-error. A diary helps this evaluation process. Over several weeks, the dosage is slowly adjusted according to the effectiveness or onset of side effects. Well-suited for long-term use, these drugs frequently cause weight gain and subtle disruptions of lifestyle, such as fatigue or malaise. A working relationship with a physician is necessary to design the most effective prophylactic program.

When considering the advisability of prophylaxis, take

into account the cost and value of headache prevention. Medication costs can easily exceed $1,000 per year. Also, the effectiveness of a specific medication frequently diminishes over time. In one study of migraine patients, only 30 percent of the patients maintained preventive benefits from their medication beyond 2 years. In addition, prophylactic medications become less effective when medications for acute treatment are overused.

There are several classes of medication which have prophylactic value in migraines or cluster headaches. For migraines, these include beta-blockers, antidepressants, valproic acid, calcium channel-blockers and methysergide. Some researchers speculate that prophylactic drugs prevent migraines by blocking a certain serotonin receptor.

In cluster headaches, the drugs commonly used are steroids (cortisone-like drugs), verapamil, methysergide (Sansert) and lithium. Appropriate dosage varies among individuals and the benefits take time to develop.

Tension-type headaches do not require prophylactic therapy unless attacks are chronic and unresponsive to acute treatment. With chronic tension-type headaches, avoid daily pain medications. When problems with sleep arise, a small dose of an antidepressant medication at bedtime can assist insomnia and diminish headaches. At times, muscle relaxants can be used to prevent tension-type headaches.

BETA-BLOCKERS

INDERAL (propranolol)
LOPRESSOR (metoprolol)
TENORMIN (atenolol)
CORGARD (nadolol)
BLOCADREN (timolol)

Several, but not all, beta-blockers have demonstrated efficacy in migraine prophylaxis. Effective dosages vary considerably and drug therapy may take several weeks before improvement becomes apparent. Small doses are initiated and increased every 2 to 3 weeks while monitoring migraine symptomatology and side effects. Using more frequent dosages throughout the day may improve results compared to longer acting, once-a-day preparations.

Side effects of beta-blockers include lethargy, lack of motivation, weight gain, decreased interest in sex, impotency, depression, decreased tolerance of exercise and low blood pressure. The heart rate slows and in rare instances heart problems may emerge.

ANTIDEPRESSANTS

TRICYCLIC ANTIDEPRESSANTS
ELAVIL (amitriptyline)
PAMELOR/AVENTYL (nortriptyline)
SINEQUAN (doxepin)

MONOAMINE INHIBITORS
NARDIL (phenelzine)
PARNATE (tranylcypromine)

SELECTIVE SEROTONIN ANTIDEPRESSANTS
DESYREL (trazodone)
PROZAC (fluoxetine)

Antidepressants help prevent migraines and promote more natural sleep patterns because they usually do not interfere with deeper levels of sleep. Beginning with low dosages decreases side effects and improves tolerability. Migraine prevention often requires a lower dosage than needed to treat depression.

The tricyclic antidepressants are the most commonly used class of antidepressants. Research has not yet documented that newer, more selective serotonin antidepressants aid migraine prophylaxis, but experience among some headache specialists supports the belief that these medications benefit migraine sufferers. Trazodone may lead to rebound headaches in sensitive migraineurs. The monoamine oxidase (MAO) inhibitors can be effective, but require careful medical monitoring.

Expected side effects of tricyclic antidepressants include sedation, constipation, dry mouth and weight gain. Rarely, they cause seizures or problems with the rhythm of the heart. Serotonin re-uptake inhibitors are less sedating, but may lead to increased anxiety and agitation. Trazodone is an exception as it is sedating. MAO inhibitors can have serious side effects associated with their use and are generally reserved for more complicated headache problems.

VALPROIC ACID (DEPAKENE)

Valproic acid is a more recent addition to migraine prophylactic medications, but has gained support from many headache specialists. Commonly prescribed by physicians as an antiseizure medication, the mechanism of action that prevents a migraine is not clearly understood. Generally, valproic acid is given several times a day. The necessary dosage is adjusted, based on blood tests. These need to be conducted periodically to insure a therapeutic level of the medication while avoiding the toxic effects of too much medication. In addition, liver tests are periodically checked as valproic acid can produce liver damage. This appears to occur more commonly in young children and only very rarely in adults.

Valproic acid is generally well-tolerated, but frequently can cause gastrointestinal upset, tremors, increased appetite and weight gain.

CALCIUM CHANNEL-BLOCKERS

VERAPAMIL/ISOPTIN (Calan or Verelan)
NIFEDIPINE/CANADA: ADALAT (Procardia)
DILTIAZEM (Cardizem)
SIBELIUM (Flunarizine)—in Canada only

Several calcium channel-blockers have demonstrated efficacy as prophylactic agents in migraines and cluster headaches. Verapamil has been studied and found to be as effective as propranolol (a beta-blocker) in preventing migraines, and is generally well-tolerated by patients. Nifedipine and diltiazem have also been reported to be successful prophylactic agents. By expanding blood vessels, calcium channel-blockers can provoke a headache in sensitive people. This generally occurs early in therapy and usually necessitates withdrawal. Short-acting formulations given in divided doses are generally more effective than long-acting once-a-day types.

Side effects frequently encountered include flushing, fluid retention, constipation, nausea, weight gain and fatigue. Periodic blood tests monitor liver function.

METHYSERGIDE (SANSERT)

Methysergide, a prophylactic medication for migraines and clusters, blocks a serotonin receptor, which probably accounts for its effectiveness. The initial small dose is increased slowly until its effectiveness can be determined.

Methysergide is associated with a rare idiosyncratic fibrosis (a type of scarring), which if left unattended, can result in serious complications and even death. Consequently, it requires careful monitoring. Many physicians recommend stopping methysergide for a planned drug holiday every 4 to 6 months to minimize its risks. Further, periodic X rays and blood tests need to be performed to assess the safety of methysergide. Adverse effects commonly noted with methysergide include gastrointestinal disturbances, drowsiness, disturbing dreams and weight gain.

Nonprescription Medications for Treatment of Migraines

Several medications not requiring prescriptions are effective in the prevention of migraines. These products are generally quite safe and have relatively few side effects. When working with a physician on headache management, however, be sure to mention the use of these products during your visit.

FEVERFEW

Feverfew is an herbal product used extensively for migraine prevention in Great Britain and throughout Europe. Available in a capsule or as a tincture from a plant in the Chrysanthemum family, the tincture has a distinctive, sometimes unpleasant taste. The dosage for migraine prevention is 1 capsule 3–4 times per day or 6–8 drops of the tincture 2–3 times per day. This dose may need to be adjusted. The full effectiveness of the treatment may not be apparent for several weeks. Side effects are few, with nausea being the most frequent complaint.

ASPIRIN

Taking 1 aspirin per day can diminish the frequency of migraines. This finding was derived from studies about the use of aspirin to prevent heart disease and stroke. Aspirin helped all three conditions. Therefore, 1 aspirin a day may be useful for many people. The only exception to this would be those allergic or sensitive to aspirin, or those on anticoagulants.

OMEGA-3-FATTY ACIDS

These food products are a special type of unsaturated fat found in certain oily fish, such as cod or sardines. In capsule form, this fatty acid is available at most pharmacies and health food stores. Taking 16 grams per day of omega-3-fatty acids decreases migraines in those studied. The major side effect is an aftertaste of fish and stomach upset. Other sources of dietary fat should be reduced while taking omega-3-fatty acids.

MAGNESIUM

Oral magnesium supplements curtail symptoms associated with Premenstrual Syndrome (PMS), including headaches. During migraine attacks, magnesium levels fluctuate. Generally, 250 to 500 mg. of magnesium per day is recommended. Magnesium may induce diarrhea if taken in excessive quantities or an individual is hypersensitive to the mineral.

Nonpharmacological Treatments for Headaches

TRANSCUTANEOUS ELECTRICAL NERVE STIMULATION (TENS)

Transcutaneous Electrical Nerve Stimulation (TENS) is a device that suppresses pain by stimulating the skin with a small electrical pulse. Nerves that register sensations other than pain are stimulated, sending a nonpain message to the spinal cord and brain. These new sensations compete with the pain sensation of the headache, resulting in less pain being registered by the nervous system. A TENS device, which looks like a beeper or small transistor radio, is clipped to a belt. The wires that connect the electrodes to the skin are arranged beneath the clothing.

The electrodes are affixed on the neck or back (they are not placed on the head), and the electrical pulse is adjusted by controls on the device. The cycle of pain is arrested by stimulation of the muscle and ultimate relaxation of the tension buildup. TENS units are effective in tension headaches and headaches resulting from mechanical factors, such as

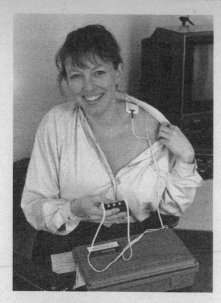

The TENS device suppresses pain by stimulating the skin with a small electrical pulse delivered through electrodes.

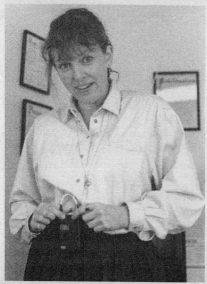

The TENS unit is clipped to a belt, and the wires that connect the electrodes are arranged beneath the clothing.

whiplash. They are safe, but require a prescription by a physician.

TRANSCRANIAL ELECTRICAL STIMULATION

Transcranial electrical stimulation uses a device that produces special electrical frequencies designed for safe application to the head. Several studies have demonstrated the value of this type of stimulation for headache sufferers. Transcranial stimulation probably enhances the release of neurochemicals like serotonin from nerve cells.

Electrodes are placed on the head and a small electrical current is applied. There is almost no feeling from the stimulation, but the individual may see a flicker of light as the current stimulates the optic nerve. This type of electrical stimulation also assists in sleep and depression.

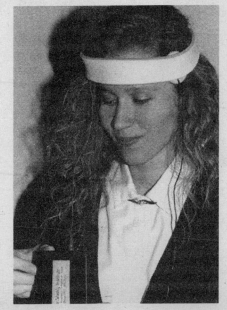

The transcranial electrical stimulation device is placed on the head to assist the individual with pain management, insomnia or depression.

ACUPUNCTURE

Acupuncture is perhaps one of the oldest treatments for headaches. Practiced throughout the world, acupuncture is used to treat attacks or to prevent future headaches.

Fine metal needles are placed through the skin in specific positions on the body. Often stimulated with electricity, the needles are left in place for 20 to 30 minutes. Excellent results with acupuncture have been reported by many individuals seeking relief from headaches. There are usually no complications from acupuncture, but it is probably wise to avoid its use during pregnancy.

ACUPRESSURE

Acupressure is the technique of applying pressure to acupuncture points rather than using a needle. Firm pressure is applied in a massage-like fashion over the selected area for several minutes. Many people find that doing this at the earliest sign of a headache can bring relief.

Conclusion

Treatment of headaches takes many forms. Medication is an important part of headache management, especially during severe headache attacks. But medication is much more effective when its use is understood as one component of a comprehensive treatment plan rather than the "answer" to headaches. Learning to balance various pharmacological and nonpharmacological treatments for headaches offers many advantages. Working in partnership with a physician who encourages safe adjunctive therapies along with appropriate medication expands the horizons for successful long-term headache care.

ACUPRESSURE POINTS

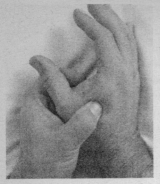

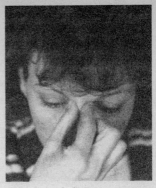

Point 1: *Apply firm pressure in the crease between the thumb and index finger. This point is often tender during a headache. Feel the release of tension after pressing deeply for 5 minutes at the onset of a headache.*

Point 2: *Apply firm pressure where the septum of the nose joins the forehead. Pressing deeply for several minutes is often effective for alleviating a frontal or sinus headache.*

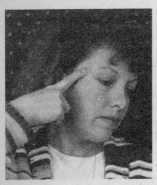

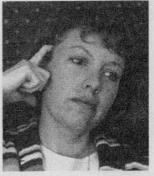

Point 3: *For a temporal headache, apply firm pressure at the tender point between the eye and ear.*

Point 4: *Apply firm pressure above the ear at the hairline for a headache localized at the side of the head.*

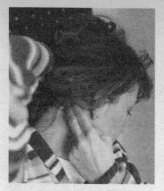

Point 5: Press firmly on the space between the ear and spinal column for a headache that originates at the back of the junction between the head and neck, but is felt in the forehead or behind the eye.

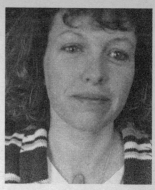

Point 6: For a bilateral headache, push down into the notch of the collarbone.

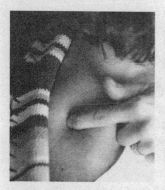

Point 7: For an occipital headache (at the back of the head), press firmly down on the tender area over the trapezius muscle (at the shoulder).

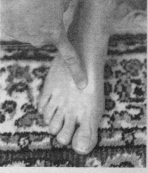

Point 8: The acupuncture point "Liver 3" is at the juncture where the bones from the first and second toes come together. Press firmly to relieve a headache, especially a migraine.

11

HEADACHES
IN CHILDREN

Studies show that a recurring headache in a child is probably a migraine. Even though anxiety may be a precipitant, rarely is it the cause of the attack. Other factors need to be investigated, such as hunger, noise, cold weather, travel, food allergy, head trauma, school stress, family disruption and alterations in lighting. Children's systems seem to be sensitive and reactive to the unique lighting of computer and television screens. In fact, moving from the dimness of a movie theater into the brightness of the sun has initiated attacks in certain children. This sensitivity can also be used to dissipate migraine symptoms. A strobe light, pulsating at a slow rate (photostimulation), has lessened the impact of an attack in children.

Prior to adolescence, 60 percent of children with migraines are boys; after puberty, males account for only 30 percent of migraineurs. Attacks in children generally last less than an hour, but some may extend over several hours, much shorter than adult migraines. Vomiting and abdominal pain may be more upsetting to the child than the actual head pain. Disruptions of sleep, including sleepwalking, bedwetting and night-terrors, are common. Research has demonstrated that migraines that begin before the age of 8 improved or stopped by age 14 in more than half the cases studied. This amelioration may be explained, in part, by the cessation of migraines in the majority of boys during puberty.

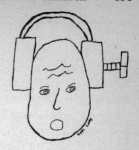

Reports indicate that a child copes with headaches much like parents do. When a child is taught not to be afraid, that a headache can be managed, he

---

Sparkles

"Hi, I'm Cindy. I'm 4 years old and I see sparkles."

Cindy's mother was beside herself with worry. She, too, sees shimmering lights, has migraines several times a month and did not want her daughter to have them. She felt guilty and afraid. She did not want to pass on to Cindy a fault, a defect, as bad as migraine headaches.

Cindy's mother sought help from a physician, who referred Cindy to a psychologist prior to starting a medication regime. Cindy responded very well to temperature biofeedback, being able to warm her fingers to 96°F within minutes. She was instructed to see the sparkles as a message telling her to warm her fingers. In this way, Cindy was able to prevent the onset of a headache. In addition, Cindy's enthusiasm over the sparkles pushed her mother into reinterpreting her own headache symptoms. She, too, learned the value of relaxation as a way to avert attacks.

or she accepts the temporary discomfort without undue up-set.

Headaches in children are a fact. Surveys estimate that by age 7, 40 percent of children have experienced a head-ache. By age 15, 75 percent report at least one episode with a headache. Paying attention to the child's complaint and offering a mild over-the-counter medication, such as aspirin or acetaminophen, helps the child feel important, cared for and acknowledged. Basically, "I count."

The Meaning of Headaches

From the child's viewpoint, the head pain may be a type of punishment. The questions to ask are:

· Where does it hurt?
· When did the hurt begin?
· How did the hurt begin?
· Does it hurt as bad as skinning your knee?

This provides a chance to discuss the pain and listen to the child's interpretation of the meaning and extent of the pain. If mild medicine does not help alleviate the pain, further investi-gation is needed.

TO A CHILD, THE HEAD PAIN MAY BE A TYPE OF PUNISHMENT.

· Do your feelings hurt as well as your head?
· Did something happen lately that upset you?
· Are you mad at one of your friends?
· How is school going?
· Have you had any problems on the school bus?

A daily headache diary is one way to help the child and parent find a link between the pain and a stressful event or internal struggle.

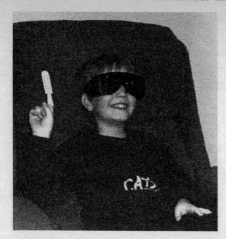

Finger thermometer and Relaxmate to help a child relax.

- Does a headache occur on days when breakfast is skipped?
- Does a headache strike after riding to school with a friend?
- Does a headache result while worrying about a date for the prom?

Also, a diary pinpoints ways to alleviate the headache. Rest or sleep may be mandated. Relaxation for 10 minutes while erasing the mind of problems and worries may wipe out pain. Biofeedback, too, is highly effective. Children learn how to warm their fingers quicker than adults, probably because a new experience is exciting and entertaining to them.

Treatment is a process of discovery. Each child has a unique headache pattern that needs to be identified. Once found, ways to divert the oncoming head pain can be practiced, such as

UNDERSTANDING WHAT PRECIPITATES HEADACHES FREES MANY CHILDREN TO PLAY WITHOUT WORRY.

eating regularly, sleeping enough and avoiding people, places and things that do not agree with one's system.

Tony is a 15-year-old sophomore in high school. The scenario for his migraines was obvious once he took the time to figure out the sequence of events. The day after a big test at school, Tony would wake up with a headache. He would sleep soundly that night because the night before the test, he would toss and turn, worrying about studying the wrong information. By planning ahead and using relaxation techniques to free the mind of upsetting thoughts, Tony seemed to be able to think better. He scored higher grades on tests. The headaches lessened to only once a month, instead of weekly.

Diet, too, is important. Chocolate, aged cheese and hot dogs push some people over the brink into a headache when there is already too much stress.

Exercise is an ideal way to release pent-up feelings and to feel better at the same time. Running, walking, biking or playing sports outside together enhances the entire sense of family and prevents headaches.

Headache Companion

I am 16 and I've had headaches everyday for the past 9 months. I'm a junior in high school and a drum major for our school band. My mom thinks that is too stressful for me, but I don't. I have to be at school by 6:30 in the morning and we practice before school until 8:17, but I really like it. I have two close girlfriends and a boyfriend, whom I've been dating for two months. My period stopped, but now it's returned and I have a normal cycle. I love opera and Mozart. I don't eat sweets or pop; I never take aspirin or Tylenol. I have one brother, three years older than me. I had another brother, but he died at age 1 of leukemia, 1 year before I was born. When I was in the eighth grade, my brother and I began fighting over what program to watch on TV. He got so mad at me that he picked up a knife and tried to stab me. I never want to see him again. My brother spent three months in a psychiatric hospital and was diagnosed as having Bipolar Disorder. He doesn't live at home anymore. I'm still afraid of him. After two biofeedback training sessions, I discovered that I didn't "make" my brother hateful. I learned how to erase negative thoughts from my mind and concentrate on the positive. My daily headaches went away. I learned how to eat right, no junk food. I make time for 20 minutes of relaxation twice a day, especially when I'm really busy. I'm getting to know me from the inside out. I used to care too much what others thought of me. Now that I like myself better, I seem to have more friends and more fun, too. But the real surprise is, no headaches.

Family Position

When a child senses, even unconsciously, that the family is disintegrating, he or she may sacrifice health to bond parents and children together. Usually the most sensitive of the family, a sick child may be an emotional barometer for the

The Barometer of Feelings

I'm 10 years old and I've had this bad headache for a week. I can't eat because I feel sick. I can't sleep because I have nightmares. We just got back from spending Christmas up north with my grandparents. Grandma has cancer and is getting radiation treatments. She's not the same, but at least she's alive; everyone expected her to die by now. Grandpa wasn't around much; he spends a lot of time with his buddies in town. His mind is somewhere else.

My mom was more upset than anyone. She cleaned the house, scrubbed the floors, even washed some of the windows. She said she's happiest when she's busy, but she didn't seem very happy. Dad wanted us to stay at a motel, not at my grandparents' house, but Mom didn't want to be separated from Grandma. She said this might be her last Christmas. My brother and I slept on the floor in the livingroom by the Christmas tree. I was so excited about catching Santa delivering the presents that I couldn't sleep. Mom and Dad didn't talk much driving back home. Mom is going to college and drives 1 1/2 hours one-way to attend classes. Dad wishes she'd stay home, but she says she needs to learn a profession. She wants to be a teacher.

My dad is not my real dad, but he seems like he is. He likes to hunt and fish and my brother and I like to go with him when he has time. He works a lot. But when he's home, we have fun. I hope Mom

> *and Dad start getting along. I don't want to go through another split-up like Mom did with our real dad.*

climate at home. A family with a problem works cooperatively toward a solution. Much like a country at war, differences dissolve and members join efforts to overcome the dilemma. When a child seems to sabotage a treatment program by refusing to

TREATMENT RESTS ON DISCOVERING THE KEY THAT UNLOCKS THE RANDOMNESS OF HEADACHES.

keep a diary or preferring to stay in bed to prevent the return of an attack, professional help may be necessary to uncover possible complex dynamics of the problem beyond that of headaches.

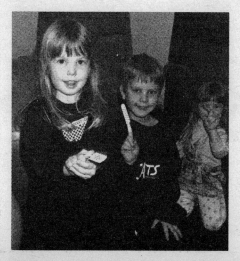

Children learn temperature biofeedback quickly, seeing the process as a game, and as a result they can divert stress rather than carry tension in their bodies.

Children need to learn responsibility for their headaches much as they do for brushing their teeth and bathing. A careful analysis of factors that probably contributed to the occurrence of an attack is part of the remedy. A realization that headaches are explainable and treatable is vital. A belief in headache control is essential for the child to gain a sense of mastery over his or her body as well as headaches.

The myths surrounding headaches begin in childhood and the facts need to replace folklore and past experiences of family members who suffer headaches. Each migraineur is an individual and each treatment plan is designed especially for that person's headache pattern. The lock-and-key mechanism of serotonin to soothe a headache may be applied on a larger scale; treatment rests on discovering the key that unlocks the randomness of headaches. Once an attack becomes predictable, it also is controllable.

In a classroom of seventeen second graders at Greenwood Laboratory School, which is associated with Southwest Missouri State University in Springfield, Missouri, fifteen 8-year-olds admitted to suffering from headaches. The following pictures by the students depict "how it feels to have a headache." Their teacher, Pauline Barker, was surprised by the depth of pain and insight the children expressed during the discussion about headaches.

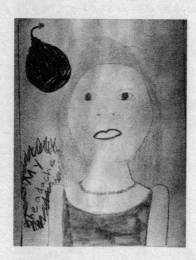

Kelly Bryan: "My headache hurts bad. A bomb is going to hit my head."

Alex W. Bethurem: "This is the cell of the headache with lightning and 2 Magnums."

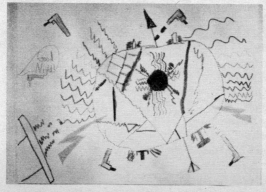

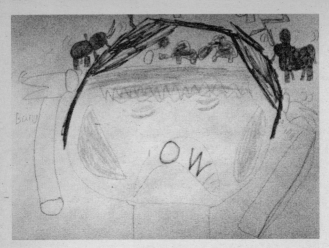

Justin Barcomb: "The worst headache feels like elephants are stomping your head."

Cara Bates: "When I have a headache, it feels like a big anvil is on my head and boxers are hitting the sides of my head. It feels so bad that I wish I could die."

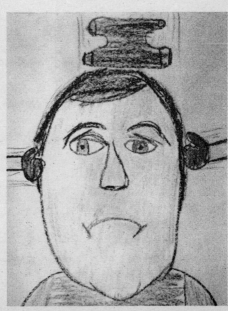

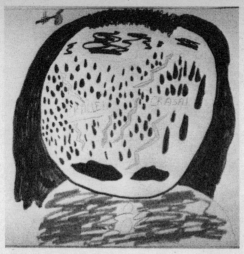

Megan Reed: "She has a thunderstorm, crackling bad inside her head."

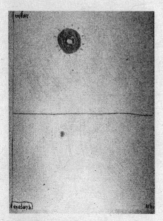

Mike Holst: "When there's a charged particle, I have a real headache. I call this a spot headache." Experts would call this an aura.

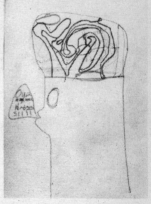

Caleb Masterson: "It feels like a bomb while lightning strikes."

Karen Ward: "My headache feels like a tight belt around my head."

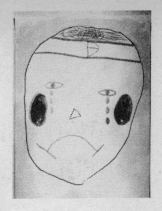

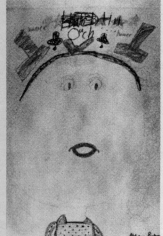

Abbey Richards: "She feels like there are hammers pounding and bells ringing on her head. Ouch!"

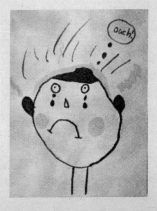

Brandon DuPree: "A bomb blew up in my head and lightning has struck."

12

CREATING A HEADACHE-PROTECTIVE ENVIRONMENT

Health care is changing. Many people desire the opportunity to participate in decisions affecting their health. Chronic conditions, like headaches, are on the frontier of this new health care partnership. An individual working with a physician has many treatment options. The medical system has much to offer, including accurate diagnosis, information, support and medications. But ultimately, the individual puts these resources into action. Many aspects of headache care are possible only through individual motivation and proper education. Forging an effective partnership with health care providers is crucial to alleviate the suffering and disability of chronic headaches.

Understanding Headaches

As a biochemical disorder, headaches affect the entire body. With a strong genetic component, headaches are a chronic condition. Headaches typically begin in younger life, become more prevalent in midlife and decline, but do not necessarily go away, with maturing adulthood. Promises of cures rarely work.

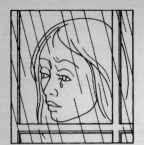

Headaches occur in response to changes in the internal or external environment, overwhelming the protective mechanisms of the nervous system. Sometimes a single factor overpowers the system, but more often, an accumulation of factors takes its toll. Many of these precipitating factors can be identified and modified to improve headache control.

For millions of people, headaches are a severely disabling illness. Recurrent attacks disrupt families and stop activities. Productivity suffers. When a migraineur can no longer work with a headache, absenteeism increases, income decreases and opportunities for promotion dim. With effective headache treatment, however, the tide turns. Individuals gain confidence and hope is rekindled.

Participating in Headache Management

Perhaps the most important vehicle for participation in headache care is a diary. Keep a record to link headache activity with changes in daily life. Learn about headache-producing factors to resolve much of the mystery and unpredictability of headaches. Avoid headache precipitants to lessen headache frequency and severity.

Engage in activities that protect the system from headaches. Regular physical exercise and a healthy diet promote well-being. Prioritize obligations to create a sense of control; "I run my life" rather than "life runs me." Value one's own needs, es-

"I RUN MY LIFE," RATHER THAN "LIFE RUNS ME."

pecially health needs, and create a headache-protective attitude of listening to oneself rather than the demands of others.

RECREATION AND RELAXATION RESTORE BALANCE AND RESILIENCE TO THE NERVOUS SYSTEM.

Restore the balance and resilience of the nervous system by establishing a regular pattern of sleep, mealtimes and recreation. Practice coping strategies and biofeedback to discover the challenges in stressful situations. Successful headache management begins when responsibility for headache control shifts from the physician to the individual.

Migraines: Marker for Other Diseases?

Migraines are an inherited neurochemical vulnerability of serotonin metabolism. Serotonin is implicated in other disease processes, such as anxiety, sleep disturbances, depression, fibromyalgia and panic disorders. Among a population of migraineurs, a higher incidence of these disorders occurs compared to those who do not suffer migraines. This has prompted researchers to theorize that migraines may be a marker for the development of other serotonin-related diseases. In fact, the natural history of migraines often involves the development of a serotonin-related disease, such as depression, in later life.

From a preventative viewpoint, control of migraines in early life not only reduces the disability of migraines, but also lessens the risk of developing other serotonin-related diseases. Learning to live a lifestyle that manages the frequency of migraines ultimately balances serotonin metabolism, decreasing the risk of developing the other diseases related to migraines.

Out-of-control migraines spawn other problems, including personal and interpersonal distress, work absenteeism and loss of self-esteem. Migraines may act as a warning that control is necessary to prevent disorders like depression. By seeking medical attention early and creating a lifestyle and environment protective against migraines, an individual is free to live again.

Rewards of
Self-responsible Headache Care

Self-responsible headache care begins with an understanding of the headache process and a willingness to become involved in managing health problems. Many important elements of headache care are under the individual's direct control. The medical system is an important resource that can assist management, but it rarely provides all the answers. Successful management of chronic debilitating headaches almost always requires modifications in lifestyle. Those willing to initiate changes will find that headache control actually becomes a prescription for self-improvement.

Creating Your Own
Headache-Protective Plan

1) Join a headache support group. If none exist in your area, there are national support groups that can provide excellent newsletters.
2) Become informed about headaches through reading.
3) Keep a headache diary and review it periodically. As understanding of headaches increases, the diary may require modifications.
4) Establish medical care and discuss headache symptomatology with the physician. Be clear and direct about your expectations.

5) Understand the proper use of prescribed medications. Disclose all medications, including nonprescription medications, to your physician.
6) Rate the effectiveness and side effects of medication. Report the results to your physician.
7) Change lifestyle habits to achieve a nutritious diet, regular exercise, smoking cessation and stress management.
8) List the goals of headache therapy, including the quality of life that is possible with headache control.
9) Seek help with problems from a physician, psychologist or a support group.
10) Recognize headaches as an avenue to more healthy living. The changes that assist the management of headaches are also good health practices.

Headaches are a complex and incompletely understood affliction. Recent advancements in the field have improved the understanding of this disorder and help validate its chemical nature. Medical treatments now provide relief by addressing the headache process rather than merely symptom control. Days of disability due to sudden headache attacks are becoming unnecessary for millions of headache sufferers.

As a chronic disorder, headaches are more than a series of acute attacks that, improperly attended, cause significant disability. Managing the chronic nature of this disorder requires a cooperative partnership with the medical system and personal motivation to be an involved participant in headache care.

Today is a hopeful time for those who have spent years being disabled by headaches. Perhaps even more exciting is a future of living more headache-free.

SUGGESTED READING LIST

Beattie, Melody. *Codependent No More*. New York: Harper Collins, 1987.

Borysenko, Joan. *Guilt Is the Teacher, Love Is the Lesson*. New York: Warner Books, 1990.

Borysenko, Joan. *Minding the Body, Mending the Mind*. New York: Bantam Books, 1988.

Cerney, J.V. *Acupuncture Without Needles*, 6th printing. West Nyack, NY: Parker Publishing, 1988.

Cooper, Kenneth H. *The Aerobics Way*. New York: Bantam Books, 1978.

Dalessio, Donald J. *How to End Headache Pain*. Phillips Publishing, 1990.

Green, Elmer, and Alyce Green. *Beyond Biofeedback*. Ft. Wayne, IN: Knoll Publishing, 1977.

Igram, Cass. *Who Needs Headaches?* Cedar Rapids, IA: Literary Visions, 1991.

Lipton, Richard B., et al. *Migraine: Beating the Odds*. Reading, MA: Addison & Wesley, 1992.

Norwood, Robin. *Women Who Love Too Much*. New York: Pocket Books, 1986.

Rapaport, Alan, and Fred Scheftell. *Headache Relief*. New York, NY: Simon & Schuster, 1991.

Saper, Joel R. *Help for Headaches*. New York: Warner Books, 1987.

Shealy, C. Norman. *90 Days to Self-Health*. New York: Bantam Books, 1987.

170   Suggested Reading List

Shealy, C. Norman. *Pain Game*. Berkeley, CA: Celestial Arts, 1976.

Shealy, C. Norman, and Caroline M. Myss. *Creation of Health*. Walpole, NH: Stillpoint, 1988.

Smith, Manuel J. *When I Say No, I Feel Guilty.* New York: Bantam Books, 1975.

FOR FURTHER INFORMATION

National Headache Foundation
(NHF): newsletter and list of
NHF physician members
5252 N. Western Ave.
Chicago, IL 60625
1-800-843-2256

HeadWay newsletter
P.O. Box 9147
Opa-Locka, FL 33054-9893

American Council for Headache Education (ACHE):
newsletter
875 Kings Highway, Suite 200
West Deptford, NJ 08096

Shealy Institute
1328 E. Evergreen
Springfield, MO 65803
(417) 865-5940

INDEX

ABOUT THE AUTHORS

ROGER CADY is medical director of the Shealy Institute in Springfield, Missouri, and specializes in the treatment of headaches and chronic pain. He received his medical degree from Mayo Medical School in Rochester, Minnesota. He is certified by the American Board of Family Practice and the American Academy of Pain Management.

As a researcher of migraines, his findings have been published in many professional journals, including *JAMA* (*Journal of the American Medical Association*), the *American Journal of Family Practice* and the *Journal of Neurology.* He is a member of the American Association for the Study of Headache, the National Headache Foundation and the American Medical Association.

KATHLEEN FARMER is a licensed psychologist and the head of the Psychology Department of the Shealy Institute. She is certified by the American Academy of Pain Management and specializes in the treatment of chronic pain and illness through biofeedback training and hypnotherapy.

As a professional writer and photographer, she has written many articles, authored *Woman in the Woods* and coauthored nine other books with her husband, Charles Farmer. She is now conducting research on the psychological characteristics of migraineurs following a variety of treatment procedures. She is a member of the American Psychological Association and the American Association for the Study of Headache.

Create Your Own Medical Library with
☑ BANTAM MEDICAL REFERENCE BOOKS

THE BANTAM MEDICAL DICTIONARY
by the editors of Market House Books

Offering the latest authoritative definitions in simple language, this exhaustive reference covers anatomy, physiology, all the major medical and surgical specialties from cardiology to tropical medicine. It also discusses fields such as biochemistry, nutrition, pharmacology, psychology, psychiatry, and dentistry.

☐ 28498-3 $6.99/$8.99 in Canada

THE PILL BOOK
7th edition
More than 25 newly approved drugs and 140 new brand names in this completely revised edition

Profiles of the 1,500 most commonly prescribed drugs in the United States: generic and brand names, dosages, side effects, adverse reactions, and warnings. Includes 32 pages of actual-size color photographs of prescription pills, as well as information on drugs with food, sex, pregnancy, alcohol, children, and the elderly.

☐ 57452-3 $6.99/$8.99 in Canada

- -

Ask for these books at your local bookstore or use this page to order.

Please send me the books I have checked above. I am enclosing $____ (add $2.50 to cover postage and handling). Send check or money order, no cash or C.O.D.'s, please.

Name _____

Address _____

City/State/Zip _____

Send order to: Bantam Books, Dept. HN 13, 2451 S. Wolf Rd., Des Plaines, IL 60018
Allow four to six weeks for delivery.
Prices and availability subject to change without notice.   HN 13 11/96

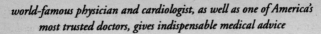

→ ISADORE ROSENFELD, M.D. ←

*world-famous physician and cardiologist, as well as one of America's
most trusted doctors, gives indispensable medical advice*

Second Opinion
Your Comprehensive Guide to Treatment Alternatives

Covering every common condition, Dr. Isadore Rosenfeld offers detailed information on why, when, and where to ask for a second opinion—and how
you can possibly avoid unnecessary surgery. ___20562-5 $5.99/$6.99 Canada

Modern Prevention
The New Medicine

In this groundbreaking book, Dr. Rosenfeld offers the latest medical
knowledge about *effective* prevention. All this is presented in the clear,
practical, and often humorous style that has become Dr. Rosenfeld's
hallmark among his millions of readers.   ___27301-9 $6.50/$8.99

Symptoms

A head-to-toe guide to all the aches, pains, and other physical "distress
signals" you may experience. In his warm, reassuring style, Dr. Rosenfeld
tells you exactly how to interpret your body's warning signs, when to seek
medical treatments, and how to stop needlessly worrying about your health.
          ___56813-2 $6.50/$8.99

The Best Treatment

The definitive guide to making informed decisions about your health.
From the common cold to cancer prevention, *The Best Treatment* gives you
the information you need to get and stay well.   ___29879-8 $6.50/$8.99

Ask for these books at your local bookstore or use this page to order.

Please send me the books I have checked above. I am enclosing $____ (add $2.50 to
cover postage and handling). Send check or money order, no cash or C.O.D.'s, please.

Name _____

Address _____

City/State/Zip _____

Send order to: Bantam Books, Dept. HN 19, 2451 S. Wolf Rd., Des Plaines, IL 60018
Allow four to six weeks for delivery.
Prices and availability subject to change without notice.   HN 19 7/95